Reporting Mental Illness in China

This book examines how Chinese-language newspapers across greater China report on severe mental illness, and why they do so in the ways they do, given that reporting in local newspapers can strongly influence how Chinese readers view the illness.

By assessing how the reporting in three leading broadsheet newspapers from mainland China, Hong Kong, and Taiwan constructs the illness, the book considers how the distinct social and political histories of the three culturally Chinese communities shape the reporting, and whether it bears out or contests the intense stigma against the illness that prevails locally. The findings can usefully encourage and inform attempts to humanise, include, and empower those with a severe mental illness across greater China and the global Chinese diaspora.

Employing a well-tested, transparent discourse analytic approach, the book also includes numerous Chinese-English bilingual news report extracts to illustrate its claims. As such, *Reporting Mental Illness in China* will be of interest to sinologists, discourse analysts, mental health professionals, and public health authorities across the globe, especially in places where there are large Chinese-speaking populations.

Guy Ramsay is a senior lecturer in Chinese language and studies at The University of Queensland in Australia. His expertise is discourse analysis in mental illness and related disorders in China and the Chinese diaspora. He published *Chinese Stories of Drug Addiction* (Routledge) in 2016.

Routledge/Asian Studies Association of Australia (ASAA) East Asia Series
Edited by Morris Low
Editorial Board: Geremie Barmé, *Australian National University*, Colin Mackerras, *Griffith University*, Vera Mackie, *University of Wollongong* and Sonia Ryang, *University of Iowa*.

This series represents a showcase for the latest cutting-edge research in the field of East Asian studies, from both established scholars and rising academics. It will include studies from every part of the East Asian region (including China, Japan, North and South Korea and Taiwan) as well as comparative studies dealing with more than one country. Topics covered may be contemporary or historical, and relate to any of the humanities or social sciences. The series is an invaluable source of information and challenging perspectives for advanced students and researchers alike.

For more information about this series, please visit:
https://www.routledge.com/Routledge-Asian-Studies-Association-of-Australia-ASAA-East-Asian-Series/book-series/SE0467

Reporting Mental Illness in China

Guy Ramsay

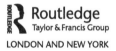

Routledge
Taylor & Francis Group

LONDON AND NEW YORK

First published 2021
by Routledge
2 Park Square, Milton Park, Abingdon, Oxon OX14 4RN

and by Routledge
52 Vanderbilt Avenue, New York, NY 10017

Routledge is an imprint of the Taylor & Francis Group, an informa business

© 2021 Guy Ramsay

British Library Cataloguing-in-Publication Data
A catalogue record for this book is available from the British Library

Library of Congress Cataloging-in-Publication Data
A catalog record has been requested for this book

ISBN: 978-0-367-54090-6 (hbk)
ISBN: 978-0-367-54995-4 (pbk)
ISBN: 978-1-003-09149-3 (ebk)

Typeset in Times New Roman
by Newgen Publishing UK

This book is dedicated with much love to Brianna Jade and Duncan Chung-Wei.

Contents

Figures

Acknowledgements

I wish to thank the following people for their generous help during the development and writing of this book: Felicity Berends, Ping Chen, Helen Creese, Wendy Jiang, Yenney Lai, Sheng-Hsun Lee, Yin Bing Leung, Haiyan Liang, Morris Low, Wai Wai Lui, John McNair, Annie Pohlman, Lara Vanderstaay, Carol Wical, Geoff Wilkes, and the reviewers of the manuscript.

1 Introduction

News media reports on mental illness have been extensively researched in the West. No systematic study, however, has examined Chinese-language news media reports on this key social issue. This book analyses Chinese-language print media reports on severe mental illness across three distinct geographical sites in greater China: mainland China, Hong Kong, and Taiwan. The book adopts a discourse analytic approach to examine how contemporary Chinese-language newspaper reports from these three settings construct the experience of severe mental illness. The book identifies the language used in reporting on it and considers how such language engages or contests salient discourses in play in Chinese societies, in particular cultural, political, and institutional discourses. In so doing, the book evaluates the degree to which these Chinese-language news reports contribute to or challenge the intense cultural stigma against mental illness in Chinese societies across the globe (Guo 2016; Kleinman, Yan, Jun et al. 2011; Ramsay 2013; Rosenberg 2018; Tang & Bie 2015).

Discourse analysts deem that people systematically construct their social worlds through the language they use (Chilton, Tian, & Wodak 2012; Galasiński 2013; Tian 2012). Their language is both reflective and constitutive of world views, social systems and practices, and power structures (Richardson 2007; Wang & Tsung 2015; Zhang 2012). Language offers a myriad of choices for expressing and communicating ideas (Galasiński 2013; Wang & Tsung 2015). Thus, the language used by speakers and writers is purposeful, often deliberate, in seeking to construct life events and experiences, such as severe mental illness, in ways that are in tune with certain attitudes, beliefs, ideologies, and intentions (Chilton, Tian, & Wodak 2012; Galasiński 2013; van Dijk 1988a, 2015). These attitudes, beliefs, ideologies, and intentions, in turn, inform salient cultural, political, institutional, and other discourses that are in play in any instance of language use (Ramsay 2008, 2013, 2016; van Dijk 1988a).

A large number of people across greater China suffer from severe mental illness, that is, functional disorders like schizophrenia, depression, and psychosis that seriously impact affected their day-to-day lives (Knifton & Quinn 2008; Rowe, Tilbury, Rapley et al. 2003; Whitley, Adeponle, & Miller 2015). The region accounts for around one-fifth of the world's population. Mainland

China, alone, has the largest number of people with a severe mental illness in the world, totalling tens of millions (Chan, Zhao, Meng et al. 2015; Zhang, Jin, & Tang 2015). At least twenty-six million of its 1.4 billion citizens have depression, making the illness "one of the most serious public health threats" on the mainland (Zhang, Jin, & Tang 2015, p. 99). Those with schizophrenia number over seven million, with a "lifetime prevalence" rate of the illness in urban areas of 0.83% (Chan, Zhao, Meng et al. 2015). The total figures are high but not surprising given the large population base. Prevalence rates are broadly in line with those in Western countries like Australia. The governments of greater China are allocating a significant amount of resources to address severe mental illness (Liang, Mays, & Hwang 2018; Patel, Xiao, Chen et al. 2016; Wu & Cheng 2017). Economic growth across the region also has produced a burgeoning middle class, who are starting to give equal weight to their mental, as well as their physical, health (Phillips, Chen, Diesfeld et al. 2013). In addition, many people emigrate from the region to join large Chinese migrant communities in multicultural countries like Australia. Here, public health bodies look to evidence bases such as the findings of this book to inform their health delivery practice in increasingly culturally diverse clinical contexts.

Severe mental illness is not a new social phenomenon in greater China. In earlier times in Chinese history, severe mental illness has been viewed as retribution for personal, familial, and ancestral moral failure, or a result of spiritual possession (Baum 2018; Ng 1990; Ramsay 2008; Yip 2007). During Mao Zedong's rule on mainland China, severe mental illness even was attributed to holding incorrect political beliefs (Baum 2018; Hsueh-Shih 1995; Kleinman, Yan, Jun et al. 2011; Tseng 1986; Xia & Zhang 1981). Nowadays, the authorities of mainland China, Hong Kong, and Taiwan, like their counterparts in the West, largely embrace a biomedical explanatory model of severe mental illness. Such an explanatory model is an integral part of an orthodox doctor-centred biomedical "belief system," as opposed to one that is more client-centred and mutually reflective, which Samovar and Porter (2001) point out

> focuses on the objective system of diagnosis and scientific explanation of disease [...] This approach emphasizes biological concerns and is primarily interested in abnormalities in the structure and function of body systems and in the treatment of disease. Adherents [...] view this model as "real" and significant in contrast to psychological and sociological explanations of illness. Disease is diagnosed when a person's condition is seen as a deviation from clearly established norms based on biomedical science. Treatment through surgery, medicine, or therapy is designed to return the person to the scientifically established "norm."
>
> (pp. 243–244)

As such, orthodox biomedical discourse is typically rationalist; syntactically complex; awash with scientific lexis and cause-and-effect rhetoric; highly attentive to objective, replicable, empirical fact; and generally dismissive of subjective intuition, emotion, and narrative, be it personal or cultural (Ainsworth-Vaughn 2003; Candlin 2001; Dixon-Woods 2001; Fleischman 2003; Galasiński 2008; MacDonald 2002; Mishler 1984; Ramsay 2008; Samovar & Porter 2001; Wodak 1996). Nevertheless, in embracing an orthodox biomedical explanation for severe mental illness, the role of the governing authorities in mainland China, Hong Kong, and Taiwan has changed from simply banishing or punishing those with the illness, to more compassionately assisting them and their families to access appropriate medical care and support. Government health bodies across greater China uniformly promote this supportive approach in their psychoeducational literature (Ramsay 2008, 2013). However, for laypeople in mainland China, Hong Kong, and Taiwan, such literature is just one source of influential opinion on severe mental illness. The general public's attitudes towards and beliefs about the illness may be equally shaped by its representation in official government pronouncements and legislation, autobiographical and literary writings, film and television productions, as well as in the news media. This book examines the discursive representation of severe mental illness in contemporary Chinese-language print media texts from three leading newspapers in mainland China, Hong Kong, and Taiwan, namely, the *People's Daily* [人民日报], *Ming Pao* [明報], and *Liberty Times* [自由時報], respectively.

This examination is distinct in employing a systematic, transparent, data-driven discourse analytic framework that integrates van Dijk's (1988a, 1998b) analysis of print media text, Fairclough's (2003, 2009, 2010) analysis of social experience and phenomena, and Shi-xu's (2014, 2015) analysis of norms, values, and scripts that most notably define Chinese culture. In this way, explicated discursive practices can be understood in terms of the salient influence of the media organisation that publishes a news text; social forces and phenomena that prevail in a geographical location; as well as overarching cultural traditions, positioning, and practices. The book also distinctly acknowledges variation and nuance across culturally Chinese societies, by examining newspaper reports from three diverse geographical locations in greater China, namely, mainland China, which has been under authoritarian Communist rule since 1949; Hong Kong, a former colony of Great Britain which was only integrated into the People's Republic of China in 1997; and Taiwan, a former colony of Japan which only democratised in the 1980s. While the book adopts a broadly critical approach to the study of discourse and frequently compares its findings with those of related studies that have been carried out in Western settings, it avoids expansively overlaying the explicated Chinese practices with those of another culture. Across the globe, the social experience of people with a severe mental illness is slowly improving, albeit amidst persisting social disempowerment and marginalisation. This book contributes to an understanding of the contemporary social experience for those in three geographical locations in greater China, by analysing the construction of severe mental illness in a leading mainstream Chinese-language newspaper from each location.

Chinese discourse studies on mental illness

In recent decades, a number of works have systematically explored how salient discourses shape Chinese texts that deal with mental illness. The first book to examine this issue is *Imperfect Conceptions: Medical Knowledge, Birth Defects and Eugenics in China* (Dikötter 1998). The book employs a cultural history approach in analysing official pronouncements on mental illness and other disabilities during the imperial times (pre-1912), the Republican period (1912–1949), and the People's Republic of China (1949 onward). More recently, but with a narrower historical focus, Baum's *The Invention of Madness: State, Society, and the Insane in Modern China* takes a similar approach "[i]n tracing a genealogy of madness from the late Qing to the Second World War" (2018, p. 182). Both books identify a pervasively negative construction of mental illness in texts and statements from the historical periods that they cover. These texts and statements portray Chinese people with a mental illness as genetically tainted. They present a threat to the healthy citizenry that must be controlled. These books note that such a construction of mental illness is in keeping with long-standing Chinese cultural attitudes and beliefs that place great value on social harmony, productivity, and patrilineal continuity. It also is consistent with eugenic teachings that carried significant weight in twentieth-century China. The books point out that leading figures and authorities of both the Republican era and the People's Republic of China drew on eugenic discourse to legitimise restrictions on the marriage and reproductive rights of Chinese people with a mental illness. Dikötter (1998) demonstrates this in a translated excerpt from a "popular booklet on family planning" that was published in mainland China in 1992:

> There are many types of mental disease, such as schizophrenia, manic-depressive psychosis and paranoia, and all have a genetic basis. The rate of occurrence among relatives of sufferers of mental disease is significantly higher in comparison to the average, and the results of research demonstrate that when both parents suffer from mental disease, 40% of their offspring will also be sufferers [...] Hence people who suffer from mental disease should not marry among themselves, since they are not only unable to live independently, but the risk of them giving birth to offspring with mental disease is also great [...] No matter whether one or both parents suffer from mental disease, they should neither marry nor reproduce when the disease is active.
>
> (p. 139)

The booklet ostensibly employs a scientific rationale, which includes statistical evidence and biomedical classificatory labels, to endorse a leading (eugenic) state policy of the time that sought to limit Chinese couples to a single, healthy child. In doing so, the text reinforces and perpetuates a key contributory factor to the intense stigma against mental illness in Chinese culture, namely, its hereditary potential. Thus, this official text, and many like it in cited in *Imperfect Conceptions* and *The Invention of Madness*, engage salient scientific, political, and cultural discourses in ways that severely marginalise and disempower Chinese people with a mental illness.

In *Shaping Minds: A Discourse Analysis of Chinese-Language Community Mental Health Literature* (Ramsay 2008), I examine how mental illness is constructed in texts that seek to counter this intense stigma against mental illness in Chinese culture. The book applies a rhetorical discourse analytic framework to contemporary Chinese-language psychoeducational texts from mainland China, Taiwan, and Australia. These texts, which seek to educate the general public about mental illness, present the preferred view of mental illness that is promoted by official health bodies and institutions, both government and private. *Shaping Minds* determines that the discursive forms of the mainland Chinese and Taiwan psychoeducational texts are largely indistinguishable. This is despite the fact that mainland China and Taiwan have quite different political and social histories. The book argues that these similarities between the mainland Chinese and Taiwanese texts cannot be attributed to discursive shaping by the professional voice of medicine. A biomedical aetiological explanation for mental illness may be hegemonically accepted by medical communities across the globe, including those in greater China (Ramsay 2008, 2013). Yet, in an apparent discursive paradox, the language of psychoeducational texts from mainland China and Taiwan is not dominated by what usually characterises the voice of the medical profession. Instead, the language of these texts gives greater voice to the "lifeworld" narrative of those with a mental illness and their families (Mishler 1984, p. 104; Ramsay 2008, p. 128). The texts also display a discursive logic that is typical of everyday talk and not of biomedical scientific rationale. Despite this greater everydayness of the mainland Chinese and Taiwan psychoeducational texts, in contrast to their Australian counterparts, their construction of mental illness does not empower the reader. This is because the authoritative voice of the institution is highly resonant in these texts. This voice prescriptively directs those with a mental illness and their families as to what they *should* do in mental illness, denying them choices and alternatives.

Shaping Minds argues that cultural norms, values, and scripts likely shape this construction of mental illness in the psychoeducational texts. The mainland Chinese and Taiwan texts temper the professional voice of medicine, in recognition that this voice could unintentionally validate widely held stigmatic cultural attitudes and beliefs that are grounded in heredity (i.e. a biogenetic transmission) (Dikötter 1998). The texts also communicate their psychoeducational message in ways that conform with interpersonal and persuasive norms in Chinese culture. Chinese readers would expect direction from those with professional expertise, rhetorically supported by everyday accounts by those with first-hand experience (Lu 2000; Ng 2000; Ramsay 2008; Shi-xu 2014). By contrast, the Chinese-language psychoeducational texts that are written for Chinese-speaking migrants in Australia give greater voice to the medical profession. This hegemonically aligns with the construction of mental illness that dominates mainstream Anglophone society. The Australian Chinese-language texts also differ from their mainland Chinese and Taiwanese counterparts in mantling their highly biomedicalised psychoeducational messages with semblances of choices and alternatives. This bears out a contemporary client-centred movement in the West that prioritises empowerment of the health consumer.

In *Mental Illness, Dementia and Family in China* (Ramsay 2013), I turn attention to personal life stories and film and television stories of mental illness.[1] The book employs a narrative-cum-discourse analytic framework to examine how salient discourses shape stories of mental illness told by those with a mental illness, their families, as well as filmmakers looking in from the outside. In this way, the construction of mental illness in the factual life stories can be compared with that in the fictional film and television accounts. A key finding of *Mental Illness, Dementia and Family* is that cultural discourse consistently shapes representations of mental illness in both the factual life stories and the fictional filmic stories. At times, cultural discourse shapes the stories in keeping with the professional voice of medicine, while, at other times, it counters biomedical discourse. Chinese cultural norms, for example, designate that the behaviours of people with active mental illness are highly transgressive and disruptive (Pearson 1996; Tang & Bie 2015). As a consequence, Chinese people with a mental illness need to be controlled. In the life stories and filmic stories, such control manifests in physical confinement in the home or in psychiatric institutions, or through pharmacological restraint by health professionals, as biomedical discourse often counsels. Cultural discourse also shapes the life stories and filmic stories in keeping with the professional voice of medicine, by accentuating the depth of disruption that active mental illness brings to people's lives. As a consequence, it is a narrative imperative for family caregivers to comply with directives from state-sanctioned health professionals. Such compliance has antecedents in Confucian teachings, where those without expert knowledge should cede to the authority of those with expert knowledge (Ng 2000).

At the same time, cultural discourse appears to countermand biomedical discourse through the low profile given to the biomedical explanatory model in the life stories. They point more to psychosocial rather than pathophysiological causes for mental illness. Pathophysiological aetiological explanations readily corroborate the long-standing cultural stigma that deems that mental illness runs in family lines. The stories told by people outside the immediate experience of mental illness, by contrast, openly point to pathophysiological, even biogenetic, causes for mental illness. Cultural discourse also appears to countermand biomedical discourse by commonly feminising family caregiving in extremely disempowering ways. In all texts, women single-handedly carry out the highly burdensome caregiving role in a selfless and resolute manner and at any cost to themselves. This is in line with traditional gender norms in Chinese culture. Biomedical discourse, in contrast, encourages family caregivers to prioritise their own well-being above that of a family member with mental illness. Only in this way can they hope to maintain their caregiving duties over the longer term. In addition, the salient influence of cultural discourse on the life stories and filmic stories is evident, in a decidedly disempowering way, through (i) the broad acceptance and, even, legitimisation of stigma against mental illness; (ii) recovery from mental illness necessitating a return to the very society that disempowers and marginalises people with a mental illness; and (iii) the self from before the onset of mental illness being romanticised as agreeable, hardworking, and normatively gendered (i.e. culturally embodied), in contrast to the self of now in mental illness, who is cast as transgressive, disruptive, unemployable, and unable to maintain normative gender roles (i.e. culturally disembodied) (Kleinman, Yan, Jun et al. 2011; Traphagan 2000).

Stigma: An Ethnography of Mental Illness and HIV/AIDS in China (Guo 2016) points out that this cultural disembodiment is central to the construction of people with a mental illness in mainland China as non-persons. Ethnographic analysis of life stories told to *Stigma*'s author by outpatients and inpatients of hospital psychiatric units identifies a common life trajectory of social rejection of the "non-person," followed by familial abandonment of the "non-human," whose illness is intractable or who is serially violent towards other family members (Guo 2016, p. 196. See also Ramsay 2013). Having lost the last line of protection and recognition in life, namely, the family, the dehumanised non-person can be institutionalised for good or justifiably murdered in a form of mercy killing (Guo 2016). Guo (2016, p. 31) states that Chinese cultural values tolerate such actions against people with a mental illness, who do "not deserve to be treated as a normal person with social face and dignity."

A chapter in the edited book *Discourses of Disease: Writing Illness, the Mind and the Body in Modern China* (Choy ed. 2016), as well as four articles in a special issue of the journal *Modern Chinese Literature and Culture* (Volume 23, Number 1) – which also is entitled *Discourses of Disease* (Rojas ed. 2011) – explores the construction of mental illness in Chinese literary writing. This question also is examined in a separate journal article by Linder (2011) and a doctoral thesis by Brassington (1996). These studies employ literary critical analytic techniques to show how Chinese literary writing makes use of mental illness for social and political critique. Four journal articles (Lan 2011; Linder 2011; Rojas 2011; Wang 2011) examine Chinese literary writing from the May Fourth period of the early twentieth century. This was a time, not long after China had become a republic in 1912, when young, iconoclastic writers wrote polemic pieces critical of the old Confucian order that had so shaped Chinese society (Linder 2011; McDougall & Louie 1997). Mental illness emerges as a potent motif in their writing. Deeply spurned and stigmatised in Chinese culture (see earlier in this section), mental illness functions as an effective trope for criticising the existing social and political order as "mad" (Baum 2018, pp. 6–7). The construction of mental illness in this May Fourth literary writing is exceedingly negative and disempowering, in line with widely held stigmatic attitudes and beliefs in culturally Chinese communities. Ironically, this is despite the fact that this literary writing had set out to criticise traditional cultural attitudes and beliefs. The writing casts Chinese people with a mental illness as subjectively displaced and alienated from their culture, society, and even their own families (Lan 2011; Linder 2011; Rojas 2011, Wang 2011). They are weak, paranoid, animal-like, and prone to sexual perversity (Lan 2011; Linder 2011; Rojas 2011; Wang 2011). They eventually die, often by suicide (Lan 2011; Wang 2011); or they recover their "sanity" and return to "the very same cannibalistic" society that had so ostracised them (Rojas 2011, p. 70. See also Linder 2011). The culturally shaped Chinese life stories and filmic stories that are analysed in *Mental Illness, Dementia and Family in China* (see earlier in this section) narrate similar outcomes in mental illness.

The pervasiveness and potency of Chinese cultural attitudes towards and beliefs about mental illness are corroborated by Brassington's (1996) doctoral research into the construction of mental illness and other disabilities in Chinese literary writing from the early Open Door reform period, up to the June Fourth incident of 1989. At this time, Chinese society was recovering from the traumatic ten years of the Cultural Revolution (1966–1976). A great deal of the literary writing from this time belongs to the "root-seeking" [寻根] genre, which looks to Chinese life on the margins and in the frontiers in search of a quintessential Chinese identity (Brassington 1996; McDougall & Louie 1997). The writing tends to focus on the unusual and the grotesque, which includes the experience of mental illness. Brassington (1996) identifies a number of negative stereotypes of people with a mental illness in the writing. They are cast as "abnormal," "bizarre," "hopeless," "animal-like," "unattractive," dangerous, and best confined in institutions, separated from the "general community" (Brassington 1996, pp. 202, 205, 209, 211, 215). In addition, people with a mental illness are considered unworthy of loving relationships and denied the right to have children. This literary depiction of mental illness, Brassington (1996) claims, is shaped by Chinese cultural discourse. Even avant-garde literary writers draw on the highly stigmatic conception of mental illness that is propagated by prevailing cultural discourse, in their social and political critiques.

More recent Chinese literary writing also uses mental illness to allegorically critique, at least through implication, social and political upheaval in China and the "historical violence" that has accompanied this upheaval (Yang 2011, p. 180). Linder's (2016) chapter in Choy's edited book and three journal articles (Linder 2011; Schaffer & Song 2006; Yang 2011) explore the construction of mental illness and its use as a trope in social and political critique in contemporary Chinese literary writing from the late twentieth and early twenty-first centuries. This writing, too, portrays mental illness in negative and disempowering ways, despite an intention to criticise Chinese cultural attitudes and beliefs and contemporary social structures. It commonly casts people with a mental illness as subjectively "fragmented," irrational outcasts (Schaffer & Song 2006, p. 5), who live both figuratively and "geographically" on the margins of society (Yang 2011, p. 187). They are sexually suspect or perverted, morally debased, and can be violent (Linder 2011; Schaffer & Song 2006). They have few, if any, "redeeming qualities" (Linder 2011, p. 301). Linder (2016, pp. 103, 117) observes that poetry may be the exception, in portraying courage in face of the intense "social alienation" and loss of "agency" and "self" in mental illness. However, such positive characterisation only extends to protagonists in this poetry, with fellow sufferers dehumanised as "uncivilized" and dirty (Linder 2016, p. 117).

Many of the mentally ill protagonists in this contemporary Chinese literary writing are women. This also is the case in the culturally shaped contemporary filmic stories of mental illness that are analysed in *Mental Illness, Dementia and Family in China*. Here, I argue that this feminisation of mental illness in contemporary Chinese films emphasises the subordination of Chinese people with a mental illness: "Being a woman in Chinese culture and having mental illness leave a person doubly subjugated due to the traditionally subordinate roles of Chinese women" (Ramsay 2013, p. 74). At the same time, Yang (2011, p. 179) maintains that the feminisation of mental illness in contemporary Chinese literary writing, like in many Western counterparts, resists the enduring and deep-seated "patriarchal" structures that control Chinese women's lives and bodies in contemporary urban and rural society. Chinese men and the patriarchal Chinese state, it seems, drive contemporary Chinese women "mad" (Schaffer & Song 2006). Yet, paradoxically, in many cases it is men who rescue these mentally ill women from their dismal fate (Ramsay 2013; Yang 2011). In this way, men retain discursive agency.

All in all, the construction of mental illness in Chinese literary writing that spans a century is relentlessly negative. Mental illness is figuratively employed to provide "imperative social insight" into periods of national political crisis in China (Linder 2011, p. 301. See also Linder 2016). However, Chinese literary writing about "madness, even if it speaks 'truth', is neither productive nor liberating" for Chinese people with a mental illness (Linder 2011, p. 301). A highly stigmatic, culturally shaped view of mental illness for the most part remains uncontested and, as a result, is reinforced and perpetuated by this literary writing in deeply disempowering and marginalising ways.

Chinese discourse studies on mental illness document a rather bleak picture of it in Chinese societies. They show that a wide range of texts drawn from the present day and the past – official pronouncements, psychoeducational brochures, personal life stories, films, and literary works – construct mental illness in highly negative and disempowering ways. Chinese cultural norms, values, and scripts appear to play a major role in shaping this representation of mental illness. Even when the intention of the texts is to resist or counter these prevailing norms, values, and scripts, the texts often contradictorily reinforce long-held stigmatic attitudes towards and beliefs about mental illness in culturally Chinese communities. This book investigates whether another highly influential but, to date, unstudied text genre, namely, print media text, constructs severe mental illness in similar ways or in ways that are more beneficial and empowering to Chinese people with a mental illness.

News media reporting of mental illness in the West

A great deal of research into news media reporting of mental illness in the West has been carried out over recent decades. Since the recognition, in the 1960s and 1970s, of the need to counter widely held negative stereotypes of mental illness in Western countries, a large number of studies have explored the construction of mental illness in news media texts. The studies believe that news media texts reflect and hold great sway over general public attitudes towards and beliefs about social phenomena such as mental illness (Anderson 2003; Georgaca & Bilić 2007; Kesic, Ducat, & Thomas 2012; Ma 2017; Nairn, Coverdale, & Coverdale 2011; Ohlsson 2018; Rukavina, Nawka, Brborović et al. 2012; Stout, Villegas, & Jennings 2004; Thornicroft, Goulden, Shefer et al. 2013; Wahl 2003; Whitley & Berry 2013; Whitley & Wang 2017). Large-scale synchronic and diachronic studies, mostly conducted in the Anglophone West, but also in continental Europe and South America, have identified a generally consistent construction of mental illness in news reports (Corrigan, Powell, & Michaels 2013). This construction is mostly negative and somewhat resistant to change over time (Huang & Priebe 2003; Kesic, Ducat, & Thomas 2012; McGinty, Kennedy-Hendricks, Choksy et al. 2016; Nairn, Coverdale, & Coverdale 2011; Rhydderch, Krooupa, Shefer et al. 2016; Stout, Villegas, & Jennings 2004). It also is gendered, usually in disempowering ways (Barnett 2005; Bengs, Johansson, Danielsson et al. 2008; Harper 2009). Whitley, Adeponle, and Miller (2015, p. 331) observe that Western news reports commonly construct mentally ill men as "fundamentally 'bad'" and mentally ill women as "sad." This negative construction of mental illness persists across tabloid and broadsheet newspapers (Clement & Foster 2008). Moreover, it persists despite wide-ranging community psychoeducational campaigns and targeted psychoeducational training of news journalists (Francis, Pirkis, Blood et al. 2004).

Studies of Western news reports on mental illness also point to their colonisation by the language and rhetoric of biomedicine (Corrigan, Watson, Gracia et al. 2005; Dubugras, Evans-Lacko, & de Jesus Mari 2011; Georgaca & Bilić 2007; Rowe, Tilbury, Rapley et al. 2003; Rukavina, Nawka, Brborović et al. 2012; Wahl, Wood, & Richards 2002; Whitley & Berry 2013). This constructs mental illness in line with commonplace physical illness, such as diabetes or hypertension. It has a pathophysiological aetiological basis that can be corrected through pharmacotherapeutic intervention, under the careful management of health professionals (Harper 2005, 2009; Ohlsson 2018). Bengs, Johansson, Danielsson et al. (2008) observe that this biomedicalisation of mental illness is more commonly encountered in Western news reports about women. Men, by contrast, are more likely to develop mental illness due to psychosocial reasons, such as work stress. As such, their mental illness has a "sudden onset," in contrast to the more "insidious onset" for women (Bengs, Johansson, Danielsson et al. 2008, p. 966). Dubugras, Evans-Lacko, and de Jesus Mari (2011), Harper (2009), and Rukavina, Nawka, Brborović et al. (2012) point out that such a construction of mental illness directly impacts on the lives of women and men with mental illness, as well as on mental illness policy formulation by Western governments and allied bodies.

The most common attribution to people with a mental illness in Western news reports is that they are menacing and to be feared (Blood & Holland 2004; Coverdale, Nairn, & Claasen 2002; Georgaca & Bilić 2007; Kesic, Ducat, & Thomas 2012; McGinty, Kennedy-Hendricks, Choksy et al. 2016; Nairn 2007; Wahl, Wood, & Richards 2002; Whitley, Adeponle, & Miller 2015). Reports portray them as commonly engaging in random acts of criminality and violence (Georgaca & Bilić 2007; Kesic, Ducat, & Thomas 2012; McGinty, Kennedy-Hendricks, Choksy et al. 2016; Nairn, Coverdale, & Coverdale 2011; Olstead 2002). Rukavina, Nawka, Brborović et al. (2012. p. 1141) state that news reporting of violence in mental illness "more often" encompasses "hetero-aggressive acts (homicide, physical assault, aggression against objects, sexually aggressive and verbal threatening)", than "auto-aggressive ones (committed or attempted suicide, self-harm)." Western news reports, at times, draw together this criminalisation of mental illness and its prevailing biomedicalisation in official circles, by endorsing the incarceration of forensic psychiatric patients in institutions as good and proper (Angermeyer & Schulze 2001; Blood, Putnis, & Pirkis 2002). In this way, "psychiatric hospitals" are conflated with "prisons" (Angermeyer & Schulze 2001, p. 473), from where people with a mental illness are "released" rather than discharged (Clement & Foster 2008, p. 182).

While this sensational facet of the experience of mental illness, at times, is real (Angermeyer & Schulze 2001; Harper 2005, 2009; van Dorn, Volavka, & Johnson 2012), it is not commonplace (Georgaca & Bilić 2007; van Dorn, Volavka, & Johnson 2012; Varshney, Mahapatra, Krishnan et al. 2016). Varshney, Mahapatra, Krishnan et al. (2016) tellingly point out that

> in order to prevent one stranger homicide, 35 000 patients with schizophrenia judged to be at high risk of violence would need to be detained [...] [E]ven if the elevated risk of violence in people with mental illness is reduced to the average risk in those without mental illness, an estimated 96% of the violence that currently occurs in the general population would continue to occur.
>
> (p. 223)

The vast majority of people with a mental illness live quite everyday lives in recovery, albeit often subject to great challenges and, at times, victimisation

(Nairn & Coverdale 2005; Rukavina, Nawka, Brborović et al. 2012; Varshney, Mahapatra, Krishnan et al. 2016). Western news reports, however, give very little attention to this everyday life in recovery (Corrigan, Powell, & Michaels 2013; Nairn & Coverdale 2005; Rukavina, Nawka, Brborović et al. 2012; Whitley, Adeponle, & Miller 2015). This is because, as Angermeyer and Schulze (2001) point out,

> It is only through spectacular negative events that mental disorders, and psychotic disorders in particular, get media attention [...] If it were not for co-occurring "newsworthy" (and usually negative) events, then mental illness would barely be a subject in the press at all.
>
> (p. 476)

As a result, Western news reports exile people with a mental illness to the margins of society, robbing them of their "social identity" (Olstead 2002, p. 625). Here, they remain, for the most part, helpless and "economically dependent on the 'rest' of society" (Olstead 2002, p. 625. See also Angermeyer & Schulze 2001; Georgaca & Bilić 2007; Knifton & Quinn 2008; Wahl, Wood, & Richards 2002).

Certainly, Western news media like to focus on the sensational (Angermeyer & Schulze 2001; Kesic, Ducat, & Thomas 2012). This is a fact of life in the current age. It, therefore, should not be surprising that news reports on mental illness are sensationalised. Such reports, however, negatively impact on people with a mental illness, by confirming and legitimising, in disempowering ways, negative and prejudiced stereotypical attitudes towards and beliefs about mental illness. A small number of studies, however, identify more enlightened Western news reporting. Coverdale, Nairn, and Claasen (2002, p. 699), while acknowledging that the New Zealand news media is overwhelmingly marked by negative reporting of mental illness, point to some positive reporting that addresses "human rights themes, leadership (e.g. director of a commune), sporting prowess or educational accomplishments." Francis, Pirkis, Blood et al. (2004, p. 545) similarly point to positive reporting in the Australian news media that addresses "policy and program initiatives in mental health [and] individual experiences of mental illness," while avoiding "stories relating to crime and dangerousness." Whitley and Wang (2017, p. 283) also identify an increasingly "positive tone" to the reporting in Canadian news media of late, with greater voice given to those with a mental illness, although reporting on crime and violence, contradictorily, is on the increase.

A vast majority of these studies of news reporting on mental illness in the West adopt a content analytic methodological approach. While very suitable for large news text corpora, content analyses inherently overlook the detail and nuance of language in use (Knifton & Quinn 2008; van Dijk 1988a). This is because the approach is "focused on revealing *what* the media say about mental illness as opposed to investigating *how* it is constituted in text" (Olstead 2002, p. 622, original emphasis. See also Kesic, Ducat, & Thomas

2012) As a result, the "exercise of power" in news reports can go "unrecognised" (Olstead 2002, p. 632. See also Harper 2005).

Olstead's (2002) discourse analysis of Canadian news reports on mental illness identifies frequent othering of people with a mental illness in disempowering ways. The reports construct subjectivities using contrastive notions of "Us," namely, the "naïve and innocent" mentally well general public; and "Them," namely, the poor, bad, "passive," and "child-like" people with a mental illness (Olstead 2002, pp. 629–630, 634). People with a mental illness, in turn, are constructed, in an apparent contradiction, as "simultaneously rational," in having the competence to successfully commit crime; and "irrational," in being "mad" (Olstead 2002, p. 630). Moreover, on the rare occasions that people with a mental illness are given a voice in these news reports, only the voices of those who are from the "socially connected" middle class can be heard (Olstead 2002, p. 640. See also Harper 2009). In the reports, they tend to have depression, while the poor suffer from schizophrenia. As a result, any positive "humanitarian content" in the reports is "organised within the structure of a dominant discriminatory narrative," here, based on class (Olstead 2002, p. 629. See also Harper 2009).

Georgaca and Bilić's (2007) discourse analytic study of Serbian news reports on mental illness also documents a discursive disempowerment of people with a mental illness. The study finds that these news reports rob them of their "social identity," connection, and value (Georgaca & Bilić 2007, p. 175). Their voice is constantly subordinated to the authoritative voice of health experts, and their illness is cast as a contagion that must be "treated and managed" by these experts (Georgaca & Bilić 2007, p. 171). The news reports construct mental illness as a homogeneous entity. There is little differentiation between the various forms of mental illness (Georgaca & Bilić 2007; Knifton & Quinn 2008; Wahl, Wood, & Richards 2002). This "consolidate[s] [...] the difference between normality and abnormality," with mental illness clearly located within the latter (Georgaca & Bilić 2007, p. 175). As such, it is readily equated to other socially marginalised ailments, such as illicit drug addiction and HIV-AIDS. These ailments, Georgaca and Bilić (2007) state, seemingly present a grave threat to the Serbian people and their nation and, accordingly, must be controlled (see also Paterson 2006).

The discourse analyses of Australian news reports on mental illness by Rowe, Tilbury, Rapley et al. (2003) and Kesic, Ducat, and Thomas (2012) also identify a subordination of the voices of people with a mental illness. This occurs even when their illness is named using a diagnostic label (Rowe, Tilbury, Rapley et al. 2003). As a result, people with a mental illness are disempowered, in that "[o]wnership of the problem is thus vested in the hands of the experts rather than ordinary people" (Rowe, Tilbury, Rapley et al. 2003, p. 684). Disempowerment also manifests in health experts being conferred grammatical agency through use of the active voice, while people with a mental illness are denied such agency through use of the passive voice (Rowe, Tilbury, Rapley et al. 2003). Rowe, Tilbury, Rapley et al. (2003), however, observe that Australian news reports on depression differ from reports on other mental illnesses by the relative absence of criminality and violence. In addition, these reports place a greater emphasis on the impact of depression on the afflicted individuals, rather than on those around them and the broader society. This impact, nevertheless, is still narrated by the authoritative experts and not by people with a mental illness themselves. This leaves these news reports, like counterpart reports on other mental illnesses, dominated by "three broad discursive repertoires – the biomedical, the administrative/managerial and the psycho-social [...] which are sometimes juxtaposed as opposing approaches, and sometimes interlaced with each other into a complex whole" (Rowe, Tilbury, Rapley et al. 2003, pp. 684, 689). Meanwhile, lay voices remain silent or are tactically coopted to "*buttress*" these discourses (Rowe, Tilbury, Rapley et al. 2003, p. 691, original emphasis).

News media reporting of mental illness in greater China

The previous section draws attention to the relative paucity of discourse analytic studies in news reporting of mental illness. The section also shows that existing discourse analytic studies are limited to Western news reports. To date, there have been no discourse analytic studies of news reports on mental illness from the developing world, including greater China. This is despite the fact that, as Zhang, Jin, and Tang (2015, p. 100) state, Chinese "news media play a pivotal role in enhancing mental health literacy." Peng and Tang (2010, p. 695) concur:

> Newspapers are one of the most important sources of health information for the public in China [...] A survey of 1,000 randomly sampled residents of Beijing showed that [...] 62.7% chose newspapers and magazines [...] as their health information source. Furthermore, 50% of health-related behavior changes were attributed to mass media.

While there have been no discourse analytic studies of news reports on mental illness from greater China, three content analytic studies have examined news reports from mainland China and Hong Kong. Yang and Parrott (2018) and Zhang, Jin, and Tang (2015) analyse mainland Chinese news reports on schizophrenia and depression, respectively. Yang and Parrott (2018) draw attention to the consistently negative reporting on schizophrenia, in line with long-standing cultural stigma. Zhang, Jin, and Tang (2015), meanwhile, point out that, while news reports on depression readily assign causal responsibility to the individual, they are

> less concerned about attaching "a human face" to [the] issue. Rather, they frequently focused on broad themes and big-picture scenarios, such as

the mounting threats of depression to a particular community or demographic group, a new government campaign to raise awareness, or new research to combine Chinese and Western medical treatment. Typical news articles utilized generous doses of facts and statistics, but, less frequently, quotes and stories from individual sufferers. When personal stories did make it into news coverage, they were often presented as patient cases with diagnostic and treatment information rather than stories with characters, plots, and affective appeals.

(p. 110)

Zhang, Jin, and Tang (2015, p. 111) trace this "phenomenon" of blaming an otherwise "invisible victim," while drawing attention to the larger social impact of mental illness, to the "collectivistic culture" and "state-controlled media system" in mainland China. These forces combine to direct blame away from, and focus concern on, the dependable and unerring party and state. Zhang, Jin, and Tang (2015), however, appear to overlook the role of Chinese cultural stigma, as described by the Chinese discourse studies on mental illness reviewed earlier in this chapter. Scambler's (2004, p. 33, original emphasis) *"felt stigma,"* that is, internalised *"shame"* or the *"fear of"* social rejection and discrimination, may discourage Chinese people from publicly speaking out about their experiences of mental illness. They tend to conceal their own or other family members' mental illness (Guo 2016; Kleinman, Yan, Jun et al. 2011; Lam, Pearson, Ng et al. 2011; Phillips, Pearson, Li et al. 2002; Rosenberg 2018; Tang & Bie 2015; Zhuang, Wong, Cheng et al. 2017). This is because public disclosure of mental illness risks great loss of social face for those with a mental illness and their family members alike (Guo 2016; Ramsay 2008, 2013; Rosenberg 2018).

In the other content analytic study of news reports on mental illness from greater China, Chan, Ching, Lam et al. (2017) analyse the use of the Chinese neologism *sijueshitiao* [思覺失調] in Hong Kong news reports that deal with schizophrenia and related psychotic mental illness. They compare the use of this quite new expression with that of its linguistic predecessor, *jingshenfenlie* [精神分裂]. This latter expression, which, in fact, is the conventional diagnostic label for schizophrenia, is highly stigmatised in Chinese culture (Pearson 1996). The newer label, on the other hand, is connotatively "neutral" (Chan, Ching, Lam et al. 2017, p. 345). Chan, Ching, Lam et al. (2017), nevertheless, caution that this apparent neutrality of the newer label may stem from Hong Kong newspapers limiting its use to reports that deal with mild psychosis. Meanwhile, they continue to use its linguistic predecessor in reports that deal with severe psychosis, where there have been incidences of violence and criminality. Chan, Ching, Lam et al. (2017) add that research suggests that changing the name of a mental illness may have little impact on long-standing stigmatic social attitudes and beliefs. Aoki, Aoki, Goulden et al. (2016), however, observe an improvement in reporting on schizophrenia in Japanese newspapers, following its renaming in 2002. The upcoming section setting out the book's approach to the analysis of Chinese-language print media reports on severe mental illness provides more detail on the existing complexity in Chinese-language mental illness terminology.

A discourse analytic approach

This book adopts a discourse analytic approach to examine how Chinese-language news reports construct severe mental illness. As noted in the previous section, discourse analysis more readily and thoroughly captures detail and nuance in the interplay between language and social phenomena (Harper 2005; Kesic, Ducat, & Thomas 2012; Knifton & Quinn 2008; Olstead 2002; van Dijk 1988a, 2015; Wodak & Meyer 2009). Fairclough (2010, pp. 132–133) represents this interplay in his three dimensions of text, discursive practice, and social practice. Text constitutes the language product, here, print media text. Discursive practice constitutes the site of, and the related conventions pertaining to, the production and interpretation of the text, here, mass media organisations and the schema that they employ in reporting the news. Social practice constitutes the social phenomenon or experience of interest and the "immediate" or "wider" social structures that define or control it, here, severe mental illness in contemporary culturally Chinese societies (Fairclough 2010, p. 132).

These three discursive dimensions inform this book's analysis of the construction of severe mental illness in contemporary Chinese-language print media texts. The book analyses the linguistic and broader textual features of newspaper reports (text) from mainland China, Hong Kong, and Taiwan (Fairclough 2010; Galasiński 2013; Richardson 2007; Tian 2012). It considers the schematic, structural, and institutional conventions of the regional media organisations that published the news texts (discursive practice) (Fairclough 2010; Richardson 2007; van Dijk 1988a, 1988b). It also takes into account the prevailing norms, values, scripts, and narratives that shape society's understandings of severe mental illness in these three geographical regions (social practice) (Fairclough 2010; Richardson 2007; Shi-xu 2014, 2015, van Dijk 1988a). The operational details of this methodology are presented in the following section of this chapter. The fundamental questions that such a methodology can help answer, however, include:

> what does this text say about the society in which it was produced and the society that it was produced for? What influence or impact do we think that the text may have on social relations? Will it help to continue inequalities and other undesirable social practices, or will it help to break them down?
>
> (Richardson 2007, p. 42)

Analysis of Chinese-language print media reports on severe mental illness

This book analyses contemporary Chinese-language print media reports on severe mental illness. The reports are published in a leading newspaper from mainland China, Hong Kong, and Taiwan, namely, the *People's Daily*, *Ming Pao*, and *Liberty Times*, respectively. These newspapers are chosen due to their wide circulations and respected reputations as mainstream local broadsheets that are less impacted by, although not wholly unaffected by, a commercialised sensational and populist agenda. The *People's Daily*, as the official messenger for the Chinese Communist Party, stands somewhat apart from its politically more independent Hong Kong and Taiwan counterparts. The reporting deals with generic severe mental illness [精神病], as well as specific disorders that the general public would readily identify as severe mental illness, namely, depression [抑郁症/ 憂鬱症], schizophrenia [精神分裂/ 思覺失調], and psychosis [精神错乱] (Knifton & Quinn 2008; Rowe, Tilbury, Rapley et al. 2003; Whitley, Adeponle, & Miller 2015). The book uses the Factiva newspaper database to source contemporary reports that name these illnesses in their headline or their lead paragraph, or in their reporting of the main event in the absence of a lead paragraph. These components represent the uppermost levels of the news text superstructural hierarchy (van Dijk 1988a, 2015). The Factiva search finds 205 reports in total, covering similar contemporary six-month time periods for all newspapers, with an additional six-month period for the mainland Chinese newspaper. The number of sourced reports is sufficient to reach saturation level in the data analysis, whereby definitive discursive trends are clearly evident (Corbin & Strauss 2008). The book analyses all of the 205 sourced reports, regardless of the extent to which they deal with severe mental illness. This is broadly in line with the rationale advanced by Wahl, Wood, and Richards (2002) in their analysis of news reports, that "every mention of mental illness, however unelaborated, communicates information about mental illness and therefore has the potential to influence public perceptions" (p. 16).

Chinese mental illness terminology is more complex than that of English. The generic English expression mental illness has four commonly used Chinese equivalents, each with its own semantic and pragmatic nuances. *Jingshenbing* [精神病] more expressly denotes severe mental illness, which is the focus of this book. The remaining three generic expressions, *jingshenjibing* [精神疾病], *jingshenzhang'ai* [精神障碍], and *jingzhang* [精障], more inclusively denote mental illness of any type, although they tend to be used where there is a greater focus on milder forms, such as anxiety disorders, obsessive-compulsive disorder, or stress response syndromes. This is especially so for the neologism *jingshenzhang'ai*, and its contracted form, *jingzhang*. They replace the Chinese characters for "illness" [疾/ 病] with those for "impediment" [障/ 碍], which is translated more idiomatically as "disorder" in this context. The linguistic change from illness to disorder stems from the intense stigmatisation in Chinese culture of severe psychiatric illness, as opposed to everyday psychological impairments (Guo 2016; Kleinman, Yan, Jun et al. 2011; Ramsay 2013). An analogous Factiva search using the three inclusive generic expressions finds that they are very rarely used in isolation in *Ming Pao* reports, and, while used in isolation more often in their *Liberty Times* and *People's Daily* counterparts, their overall numbers are far lower than those for expressions denoting severe mental illness, with which this book is concerned.

Further terminological complexity arises with the Chinese expressions for schizophrenia, namely, *jingshenfenlie* [精神分裂] and *sijueshitiao* [思覺失調]. As noted earlier on in the section on news media reporting of mental illness in greater China, the latter expression is a neologism coined to counter the intense stigma in Chinese culture against the conventional diagnostic label, *jingshenfenlie* (Chan, Ching, Lam et al. 2017; Pearson 1996). Chan, Ching, Lam et al. (2017) state that the newer label is especially used to denote first-episode psychotic illness. It, therefore, could be translated as psychosis, rather than schizophrenia. Taking into account the developmental origins of the neologism, this book chooses to translate it as schizophrenia. However, translating it as psychosis would not impact the analysis and findings of the ensuing chapters, since they show that the newspaper reports construct *jingshenfenlie* and *sijueshitiao* in identical ways. The two Chinese expressions for depression, namely, *yiyuzheng* [抑郁症] and *youyuzheng* [憂鬱症], are functionally synonymous and merely reflect regional differences in lexis.

The analysis proceeds from the premise that "mental illness and thus, those who are defined as mentally ill, are constituted" in texts "through particular organised discourses" (Olstead 2002, p. 622). The discourse analytic methodology that this book employs in its analysis of contemporary Chinese-language print media text primarily draws on the approaches of van Dijk (1988a, 1988b), Fairclough (2003, 2009, 2010), and Shi-xu (2014, 2015). Doing so enables the discursive features and strategies that characterise the news texts to be identified, examined, and assessed in terms of their genre, namely print media text; their sites of production, namely, media organisations in mainland China, Hong Kong, and Taiwan; as well as their social and cultural positioning and status.

Van Dijk (1988a, 1988b) lays out a systematic discourse analytic framework for the analysis of print mass media text. This well-tested framework recognises that the hierarchical organisation of topics in a news text is discursively significant. Meaning is not presented in a haphazard way, but is ordered and structured

in accordance with the hierarchy of journalistic newsworthiness: high-level topics come first in the linear organization of the text. The hierarchy is governed by such major controlling factors as recency (the more recent, the more important) and impact (effects come before causes, global facts before details).

(Duszac 1991, p. 506)

As a result, the reporting of topics early on or later on in a news text is discursively significant. Van Dijk (1988b) states that this ordering of information bestows a distinct schematic superstructure on news texts. This superstructure is relatively consistent across geographical settings (van Dijk 1988a, 1988b). The highest governing topic is expressed in the headline and the lead paragraph, when present. Accordingly, the headline and lead represent the uppermost, and, so, the most prominent, levels of a news text's superstructural hierarchy (Kesic, Ducat, & Thomas 2012; Olstead 2002; Sandby-Thomas 2014). These highest-level superstructural categories are followed by the news story, which typically describes an episode that is comprised of a main event and its consequences; the background, which can encompass recent contextual and historical backdrops to what is reported in the main event; as well as comments made up of verbal reactions to the main event by protagonists and other social actors, together with posited expectations or evaluations about what has occurred (van Dijk 1988b). Not all news texts contain all of these superstructural categories. In addition, the absence of a superstructural category, in itself, can be significant.

This book's analysis similarly identifies the superstructural hierarchy of the Chinese-language news texts under study and the topics expressed within. Higher-level meanings are deemed to be more prominent and newsworthy than those located in the lower levels of the news text superstructural hierarchy. The finer linguistic features that comprise a news text also gain prominence by way of their location in the news text superstructural hierarchy. These discursively informative features can include word choice, word order, syntax, metaphor use, clause choice, clause and text arrangement, statistical and scientific substantiation, meaning and vocal prominence, amongst others (Chilton, Tian, & Wodak 2012; Fairclough 2003, 2009; Olstead 2002; Richardson 2007; Rowe, Tilbury, Rapley et al. 2003; Tian 2015; van Dijk 1988a, 1988b, 2009, 2015; van Leeuwen 2007, 2009; Wodak 2014). The analysis considers that anything that is supposed, implied, mitigated, or left out of a news text is just as important as what is made explicit (Kesic, Ducat, & Thomas 2012; Richardson 2007; van Dijk 1988a, 1988b, 2009, 2015). A news text can selectively use these features to construct or affirm racial, ethnic, gender, age, and socioeconomic identities or social relationships, celebrating in-groups and maligning outgroups (Harper 2009; Richardson 2007; van Dijk 1988a, 2000, 2014, 2015; Whitley, Adeponle, & Miller 2015). This may bear out the power of a media organisation and its attendant commercial or political agenda (Fairclough 2010; Richardson 2007; van Dijk 1988a, 2015). It also may bear out cultural norms, values, and scripts, or government policy and dictates (Fairclough 2010; Richardson 2007; Ramsay 2013, 2016; Shi-xu 2014, 2015; Tian 2012; van Dijk 1988a, 2015). These discursive repertoires may intertextually bind a news text to past and present texts from other genres, such as those discussed in the earlier section on Chinese discourse studies on mental illness (Chilton, Tian, & Wodak 2012; Fairclough 2003, 2009; Galasiński 2013; Reisigl & Wodak 2009).

The interplay between text, discursive practice, and social practice may be partially or wholly supportive or subversive, and may manifest across different texts in complementary or conflicting ways (Fairclough 2003; Wodak & Meyer 2009). Accordingly, the Chinese-language news texts that are analysed in this book may "sustain and reproduce the social status quo" in relation to severe mental illness (Angermuller, Maingueneau, & Wodak 2014, p. 362). On the other hand, they may resist and challenge it, creating a "counter-discourse" (Wang 2015, p. 128. See also Tian 2012). The resulting discursive practice is determined by the organisational setting of text production, here, three print media firms in three geographical locations; and the wider sociocultural environment. A print media firm may be especially motivated by a market imperative or political agenda. Equally, how a society views or construes a phenomenon or experience may be heavily shaped by prevailing cultural norms, values, and scripts. Shi-xu (2014, p. 21) points to the importance of such norms, values, and scripts in the discursive domain, given that "human discourses are sites of cultural contestation, cooperation and transformation" (see also Galasiński 2008; Paterson 2007). Shi-xu (2014, 2015) contends that this is particularly so for Chinese discourse. This is because of the prominent role, in Chinese discourse, of cultural phenomena such as:

- social and communicative "harmony."
- social "face."
- the voice of "authority," in particular, "social position," "moral character," "entrepreneurial success," "artistic accomplishment," and "expert knowledge."
- the voice of the everyday citizen.
- state "nationalism."
- a pragmatic and collective approach to *"problem-solving."*

(Shi-xu 2014, pp. 11–107, original emphasis)

The Chinese discourse studies on mental illness that are discussed earlier on in this chapter attest to this, drawing attention to the role of Chinese cultural phenomena in shaping the construction of mental illness in official pronouncements, psychoeducational brochures, personal life stories, films, and literary works. The analysis in this book similarly calls attention to the expression of cultural phenomena, in addition to political, institutional, and other phenomena, in Chinese-language news reports on severe mental illness.

Figure 1.1 below diagrammatically outlines this analytic approach to be employed in the ensuing chapters of this book.

Thus, analysis of a Chinese-language news report on severe mental illness proceeds from its superstructural hierarchy, whereby the headline constitutes the highest level of this hierarchy, while comments typically, but not necessarily, constitute the lowest level. The analysis successively identifies the salient semantic and finer linguistic features that characterise each component of the news text's superstructural hierarchy, starting with the headline, as

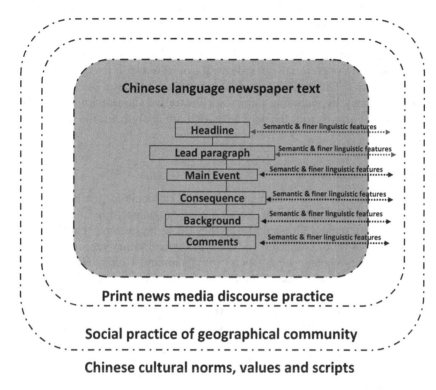

Figure 1.1 Analysis of Chinese-language news reports on severe mental illness.

the highest-level component, and then working through all of the succeeding schematic components. The semantic and finer linguistic features may encompass, for example, quotes from named leading authorities, which grammatically prioritise them as agents. This adds credibility to the claims made in the news report, a key concern for media organisations. At the same time, the voice of those with a severe mental illness is necessarily subordinated. Doing so bears out and legitimates the intense stigma towards them in the local community. Disempowering and marginalising social practices and phenomena of this kind, in turn, are shaped by long-standing norms, values, and scripts in Chinese culture, which cast people with a severe mental illness as unwanted, unproductive non-persons (Baum 2018; Guo 2016).

By adopting this systematic and integrated approach to the analysis of Chinese-language print media reports on severe mental illness, the book aims to show how they are shaped by the media organisations and culturally Chinese societies in which they are produced. It also aims to show how these texts construct and assign identities to people with a severe mental illness and how they position them in broader society. In so doing, it will ascertain whether the texts disempower and marginalise people with a severe mental illness, as it has been shown texts from other genres do; or whether they differ and challenge and confront the intense cultural stigma against these people. Such analysis is necessarily interpretative (Richardson 2007; van Dijk 2015; You, Chen, & Hong 2012). Chilton, Tian and Wodak (2012, p. 6) stress that interpretative discourse analytic endeavours of this type "must be explicit and transparent." This book attempts to maintain a high level of explicitness and transparency by including numerous illustrative Chinese-English bilingual examples, drawn from the news texts that are analysed in the upcoming chapters.

Summary of chapters

This chapter has set out the background to and rationale for the book's discourse analytic examination of how Chinese-language print media texts construct severe mental illness and why they do so in the ways that they do. Chapters 2, 3, 4, and 5 describe and analyse contemporary reports in three leading Chinese-language newspapers from mainland China, Hong Kong, and Taiwan. While all three geographical settings have culturally Chinese communities, each has its own unique social and political histories. This can impact how their local newspapers report on severe mental illness.

Chapter 2 outlines past and current statuses of severe mental illness in mainland China, Hong Kong, and Taiwan, citing relevant contemporary statistics. The chapter introduces the three Chinese-language newspapers whose reports on severe mental illness are analysed in the book, namely, the *People's Daily* from mainland China, *Ming Pao* from Hong Kong, and *Liberty Times* from Taiwan. In doing so, it points out how the choice of these three newspapers stems from their standings as leading, mainstream, locally owned broadsheets. The chapter further lists and compares the defining parameters for each of the newspapers' reports on severe mental illness. This critically includes the specific illnesses that they report on, as well as the emergent wider themes.

Organised around the recurrent themes of crime and social wrongdoing, celebrity and everyday life experience, orthodox biomedicine, and political gain and activism, Chapters 3, 4, and 5 systematically contextualise and analyse the reports on severe mental illness in the three Chinese-language newspapers. They do so by adopting the discourse analytic approach set out in this introductory chapter. Each theme-based chapter identifies and evaluates the extent to which, how, and why the reports variably disempower (or liberate), marginalise (or normalise), and dehumanise (or humanise) those with a severe mental illness, by

- sensationalising their illness.
- essentialising and gendering their subjectivities and life experiences.
- prioritising the voices of those in authority or family caregivers over their own.
- positioning them adversely vis-à-vis mentally well citizens.

- blaming them for their illness.
- privileging those with "palatable" medical diagnoses.

Each chapter indicates how such reporting selectively bears out or counters dominant cultural, political, and biomedical narratives circulating in a geographical community. The chapters further conclude whether doing so detrimentally validates a lay reader's existing "habits of mind" or "sets of fixed assumptions and expectations" in relation to severe mental illness; or magnanimously challenges and, so, potentially transforms them in ways that are "more inclusive, discriminating, open, reflective, and emotionally able to change" (Gibson & Jacobson 2018, p. 187). As this introductory chapter clearly documents, the prevailing habits of mind in culturally Chinese communities to date remain distinctly stigmatic and highly problematic for those with a severe mental illness.

Chapter 6, the book's concluding chapter, draws together the findings of Chapters 2 to 5, identifying shared trends and unique differences in the reporting on severe mental illness in the three Chinese-language newspapers. The chapter looks to wider cultural narratives, political systems, and institutional priorities to explain these trends and differences. It also compares and contrasts them with those that characterise analogous Western reporting, as detailed in this introductory chapter. Chapter 6 additionally points out the nascent tensions and contradictions that mark the reporting in the three Chinese-language newspapers. This, together with the book's wider findings, forms the basis for recommendations to encourage more compassionate, inclusive, humane, and empowering reporting on severe mental illness in newspapers across greater China and the global Chinese diaspora.

Note

1 Related work on Chinese life stories of mental illness also can be found in these two journal articles: Ramsay (2009) and Ramsay (2010).

References

Ainsworth-Vaughn, N. (2003). The discourse of medical encounters. In D. Schiffrin, D. Tannen, & H. E. Hamilton (Eds.) *The handbook of discourse analysis* (pp. 453–469). Oxford: Blackwell.

Anderson, M. (2003). "One flew over the psychiatric unit": Mental illness and the media. *Journal of Psychiatric and Mental Health Nursing, 10*(3), 297–306.

Angermeyer, M. C., & Schulze, B. (2001). Reinforcing stereotypes: How the focus on forensic cases in news reporting may influence public attitudes towards the mentally ill. *International Journal of Law and Psychiatry, 24*(4), 469–486.

Angermuller, J., Maingueneau, D., & Wodak, R. (2014). Critical approaches: Introduction. In J. Angermuller, D. Maingueneau, & R. Wodak (Eds.), *Discourse Studies reader: Main currents in theory and analysis* (pp. 359–364). Amsterdam: John Benjamins.

Aoki, A., Aoki, Y., Goulden, R., Kasai, K., Thornicroft, G., & Henderson, C. (2016). Change in newspaper coverage of schizophrenia in Japan over 20-year period. *Schizophrenia Research, 175*(1–3), 193–197.

Barnett, B. (2005). Perfect mother or artist of obscenity? Narrative and myth in a qualitative analysis of press coverage of the Andrea Yates murders. *Journal of Communication Inquiry, 29*(1), 9–29.

Baum, E. (2018). *The invention of madness: State, society, and the insane in modern China*. Chicago: University of Chicago Press.

Bengs, C., Johansson, E., Danielsson, U., Lehti, A., & Hammarström, A. (2008). Gendered portraits of depression in Swedish newspapers. *Qualitative Health Research, 18*(7), 962–973.

Blood, R. W., Putnis, P., & Pirkis, J. (2002). Mental-illness news as violence: A news frame analysis of the reporting and portrayal of mental health and illness in Australian media. *Australian Journal of Communication, 29*(2), 59–82.

Blood, W., & Holland, K. (2004). Risky news, madness and public crisis. *Journalism, 5*(3), 323–342.

Brassington, C. (1996). *The portrayal of disability in contemporary Chinese literature and its relationship to perceptions of and attitudes towards people with disabilities in contemporary Chinese society: An investigative study*. [Doctoral dissertation. St Lucia, QLD: University of Queensland].

Candlin, C. N. (2001). Medical discourse as professional and institutional action: Challenges to teaching and researching languages for special purposes. In M. Bax, & C. J. Zwart (Eds.) *Reflections on language and language learning: In honour of Arthur Van Essen* (pp. 185–207). Amsterdam: John Benjamins.

Chan, K. Y., Zhao, F., Meng, S., Demaio, A. R., Reed, C., Theodoratou, E., Campbell, H., Wang, W., & Rudan, I. (2015). Prevalence of schizophrenia in China between 1990 and 2010. *Journal of Global Health, 5*(1), 1–8.

Chan, S. K. W., Ching, E. Y. N., Lam, K. S. C., So, H., Hui, C. L. M., Lee, E. H. M., Chang, W. C., & Chen, E. Y. H. (2017). Newspaper coverage of mental illness in Hong Kong between 2002 and 2012: Impact of introduction of a new Chinese name of psychosis. *Early Intervention in Psychiatry*, 11(4), 342–344.

Chilton, P., Tian, H., & Wodak, R. (2012). Reflections on discourse and critique in China and the West. In P. Chilton, H. Tian, & R. Wodak (Eds.), *Discourse and socio-political transformations in contemporary China* (pp. 1–18). Amsterdam: John Benjamins.

Choy, H. Y. F. (Ed.) (2016). *Discourses of disease: Writing illness, the mind and the body in modern China*. Leiden: Brill.

Clement, S., & Foster, N. 2008. Newspaper reporting on schizophrenia: A content analysis of five national newspapers at two time points. *Schizophrenia Research, 98*(1), 178–183.

Corbin, J. M., & Strauss, A. L. (2008). *Basics of qualitative research: Techniques and procedures for developing grounded theory* (3rd ed.). Thousand Oaks, CA: SAGE.

Corrigan, P. W., Powell, K. J., & Michaels, P. J. (2013). The effects of news stories on the stigma of mental illness. *Journal of Nervous and Mental Disease, 201*(3), 179–182.

Corrigan, P. W., Watson, A. C., Gracia, G., Slopen, N., Rasinski, K., & Hall, L. L. (2005). Newspaper stories as measures of structural stigma. *Psychiatric Services, 56*(5), 551–556.

Coverdale, J., Nairn, R., & Claasen, D. (2002). Depictions of mental illness in print media: A prospective national sample. *Australasian Psychiatry, 36*(5), 697–700.

Dikötter, F. (1998). *Imperfect conceptions: Medical knowledge, birth defects and eugenics in China.* London: Hurst & Co.

Dixon-Woods, M. (2001). Writing wrongs? An analysis of published discourses about the use of patient information leaflets. *Social Science and Medicine, 52*(9), 1417–1432.

Dubugras, M. T. B., Evans-Lacko, S., & de Jesus Mari, J. 2011. A two-year cross-sectional study on the information about schizophrenia divulged by a prestigious daily newspaper. *Journal of Nervous and Mental Disease, 199*(9), 659–665.

Duszac, A. (1991). Schematic and topical categories in news story reconstruction. *Text, 11*(4), 503–522.

Fairclough, N. (2003). *Analysing discourse: Textual analysis for social research.* Routledge.

Fairclough, N. (2009). A dialectical-relational approach to Critical Discourse Analysis in social research. In R. Wodak, & M. Meyer (Eds.), *Methods of critical discourse analysis* (pp. 162–186). London: SAGE.

Fairclough, N. (2010). *Critical discourse analysis: The critical study of language.* Harlow, UK: Longman.

Fleischman, S. (2003). Language and medicine. In D. Schiffrin, D. Tannen, & H. E. Hamilton (Eds.), *The handbook of discourse analysis* (pp. 470–502). Oxford: Blackwell.

Francis, C., Pirkis, J., Blood, R. W., Dunt, D., Burgess, P., Morley, B., Stewart, A., & Putnis, P. (2004). The portrayal of mental health and illness in Australian non-fiction media. *Australian and New Zealand Journal of Psychiatry, 38*(7), 541–546.

Galasiński, D. (2008). *Men's discourses of depression.* London: Palgrave Macmillan.

Galasiński, D. (2013). *Fathers, fatherhood and mental illness: A discourse analysis of rejection.* London: Palgrave Macmillan.

Georgaca, E., & Bilić, B. (2007). Representations of "mental illness" in Serbian newspapers: A critical discourse analysis. *Qualitative Research in Psychology, 4*(1), 167–186.

Gibson, C., & Jacobson, T. (2018). Habits of mind in an uncertain information world. *Reference and User Services Quarterly, 57*(3), 183–192.

Guo, J. (2016). *Stigma: An ethnography of mental illness and HIV/AIDS in China.* Hackensack, NJ: World Century.

Harper, S. (2005). Media, madness and misrepresentation: Critical reflections on anti-stigma discourse. *European Journal of Communication, 20*(4), 460–483.

Harper, S. (2009). *Madness, power and the media: Class, gender and race in popular representations of mental distress.* Basingstoke, UK: Palgrave Macmillan.

Hsueh-Shih, C. (1995). Development of mental health systems and care in China: From the 1940s through the 1980s. In T. Lin, W. Tseng, & E. Yeh (Eds.), *Chinese society and mental health* (pp. 315–325). Hong Kong: Oxford University Press.

Huang, B., & Priebe, S. (2003). Media coverage of mental health care in the UK, USA and Australia. *Psychiatric Bulletin, 27*(9), 331–333.

Kesic, D., Ducat, L. V., & Thomas, S. D. (2012). Using force: Australian newspaper depictions of contacts between the police and persons experiencing mental illness. *Australian Psychologist, 47*(4), 213–223.

Kleinman, A., Yan, Y., Jun, J., Lee, S., Zhang, E., Pan, T., Wu, F., & Guo, J. (2011). *Deep China: The moral life of the person: What anthropology and psychiatry tell us about China today.* Berkeley, CA: University of California Press.

Knifton, L., & Quinn, N. (2008). Media, mental health and discrimination: A frame of reference for understanding reporting trends. *International Journal of Mental Health Promotion, 10*(1), 23–31.

Lam, M. M. L., Pearson, V., Ng, R. M. K., Chiu, C. P .Y., Law, C. W., & Chen, E. Y. H. (2011). What does recovery from psychosis mean? Perceptions of young first-episode patients. *International Journal of Social Psychiatry, 57*(6), 580–587.

Lan, F. (2011). From the de-based literati to the de-based intellectual: A Chinese hypochondriac in Japan. *Modern Chinese Literature and Culture, 23*(1), 105–132.

Liang, D., Mays, V., & Hwang, W. (2018). Integrated mental health services in China: Challenges and planning for the future. *Health Policy and Planning, 33*(1), 107–122.

Linder, B. (2011). Trauma and truth: Representations of madness in Chinese literature. *Journal of Medical Humanities, 32*(4), 291–303.

Linder, B. (2016). Metaphors unto themselves: Mental illness poetics and narratives in contemporary Chinese poetry. In H. Y. F. Choy (Ed.), *Discourses of disease: Writing illness, the mind and the body in modern China* (pp. 90–122). Leiden: Brill.

Lu, X. (2000). The influence of classical Chinese rhetoric on contemporary Chinese political communication and social relations. In D. R. Heisey (Ed.), *Chinese perspectives in rhetoric and communication* (pp. 3–24). Stamford: Ablex.

Ma, Z. (2017). How the media cover mental illnesses: A review. *Health Education, 117*(1), 90–109.

MacDonald, M. N. (2002). Pedagogy, pathology and ideology: The production, transmission and reproduction of medical discourse. *Discourse and Society, 13*(4), 447–467.

McDougall, B., & Louie, K. (1997). *The literature of China in the twentieth century.* London: Hurst & Co.

McGinty, E. E., Kennedy-Hendricks, A., Choksy, S., & Barry, C. L. (2016). Trends in news media coverage of mental illness in the United States: 1995–2014. *Health Affairs, 35*(6), 1121–1129.

Mishler, E. G. (1984). *The discourse of medicine: Dialectics of medical interviews.* Norwood: Ablex.

Nairn, R. G. (2007). Media portrayals of mental illness, or is it madness? A review. *Australian Psychologist, 42*(2), 138–146.

Nairn, R. G., & Coverdale, J. H. (2005). People never see us living well: An appraisal of the personal stories about mental illness in a prospective print media sample. *Australian and New Zealand Journal of Psychiatry, 39*(4), 281–287.

Nairn, R., Coverdale, S., & Coverdale, J. H. (2011). A framework for understanding media depictions of mental illness. *Academic Psychiatry, 35*(3), 202–206.

Ng, R. M. (2000). The influence of Confucianism on Chinese conceptions of power, authority, and the rule of law. In D. R. Heisey (Ed.), *Chinese perspectives in rhetoric and communication* (pp. 45–56). Stamford: Ablex.

Ng, V. W. (1990). *Madness in late imperial China: From illness to deviance.* London: University of Oklahoma Press.

Ohlsson, R. (2018). Public discourse on mental health and psychiatry: Representations in Swedish newspapers. *Health: An Interdisciplinary Journal for the Social Study of Health, Illness and Medicine, 22*(3), 298–314.

Olstead, R. (2002). Contesting the text: Canadian media depictions of the conflation of mental illness and criminality. *Sociology of Health and Illness, 24*(5), 621–643.

Patel, V., Xiao, S., Chen, H., Hanna, F., Jotheeswaran, A. T., Luo, D., Parikh, R., Sharma, E., Usmani, S., Yu, Y., Druss, B. G., & Saxena, S. (2016). The magnitude of and health system responses to the mental health treatment gap in adults in India and China. *The Lancet, 388*(10063), 3074–3084.

Paterson, B. (2006). Newspaper representations of mental illness and the impact of the reporting of "events" on social policy: The "framing" of Isabel Schwarz and Jonathan Zito. *Journal of Psychiatric and Mental Health Nursing, 13*(3), 294–300.

Paterson, B. (2007). A discourse analysis of the construction of mental illness in two UK newspapers from 1985–2000. *Issues in Mental Health Nursing, 28*(10), 1087–1103.

Pearson, V. (1996). The Chinese equation in mental health policy and practice. *International Journal of Law and Psychiatry, 19*(3/4), 437–458.

Peng, W., & Tang, L. (2010). Health content in Chinese newspapers. *Journal of Health Communication, 15*(7), 695–711.

Phillips, M., Chen, H., Diesfeld, K., Xie, B., Cheng, H., Mellsop, G., & Liu, X. (2013). China's new mental health law: Reframing involuntary treatment. *American Journal of Psychiatry, 170*(6), 588–591.

Phillips, M., Pearson, V., Li, F. F., Xu, M. J., & Yang, L. (2002). Stigma and expressed emotion: A study of people with schizophrenia and their family members in China. *British Journal of Psychiatry, 181*(6), 488–493.

Ramsay, G. (2008). *Shaping minds: A discourse analysis of Chinese-language community mental health literature.* Amsterdam: John Benjamins.

Ramsay, G. (2009). Chinese mental illness narratives: Controlling the spirit. *Communication and Medicine, 6*(2), 189–198.

Ramsay, G. (2010). Mainland Chinese family caregiver narratives in mental illness: Disruption and continuity. *Asian Studies Review, 34*(1), 83–103.

Ramsay, G. (2013). *Mental illness, dementia and family in China.* London: Routledge.

Ramsay, G. (2016). *Chinese stories of drug addiction: Beyond the opium dens.* New York: Routledge.

Reisigl, M., & Wodak, R. (2009). The Discourse-Historical Approach (DHA). In R. Wodak, & M. Meyer (Eds.), *Methods of critical discourse analysis* (pp. 87–121). London: SAGE.

Rhydderch, D., Krooupa, A. M., Shefer, G., Goulden, R., Williams, P., Thornicroft, A., Rose, D., Thornicroft, G., & Henderson, C. (2016). Changes in newspaper coverage of mental illness from 2008 to 2014 in England. *Acta Psychiatrica Scandinavica, 134*(Suppl. 446), 45–52.

Richardson, J. E. (2007). *Analysing newspapers: An approach from Critical Discourse Analysis.* New York: Palgrave Macmillan.

Rojas, C. (2011). Of canons and cannibalism: A psycho-immunological reading of "Diary of a Madman." *Modern Chinese Literature and Culture, 23*(1), 47–76.

Rosenberg, A. (2018, June 18). Hiding my mental illness from my Asian family almost killed me: The silent shame of having a mental illness in a Chinese family. *Vox.* www.vox.com/first-person/2018/6/18/17464574/asian-chinese-community-mental-health-illness

Rowe, R., Tilbury, F., Rapley, M., & O'Ferrall, I. (2003). "About a year before the breakdown I was having symptoms": Sadness, pathology and the Australian newspaper media. *Sociology of Health and Illness, 25*(6), 680–696.

Rukavina, T. V., Nawka, A., Brborović, O., Jovanović, N., Kuzman, M. R., Nawková, L., Bednárová, B., Žuchová, S., Hrodková, M., & Lattova, Z. (2012). Development of the PICMIN (picture of mental illness in newspapers): Instrument to assess mental illness stigma in print media. *Social Psychiatry and Psychiatric Epidemiology, 47*(7), 1131–1144.

Samovar, L. A., & Porter, R. E. (2001). *Communication between cultures*. Belmont, CA: Wadsworth/Thomson Learning.

Sandby-Thomas, P. (2014). "Stability overwhelms everything": Analysing the legitimating effect of the stability discourse since 1989. In Q. Cao, H. Tian, & P. A. Chilton (Eds.), *Discourse, politics and media in contemporary China* (pp. 47–76). Amsterdam: John Benjamins.

Scambler, G. (2004). Re-framing stigma: Felt and enacted stigma and challenges to the sociology of chronic and disabling conditions. *Social Theory and Health, 2*(1), 29–46.

Schaffer, K., & Song X. (2006). Writing beyond the wall: Translation, cross-cultural exchange and Chen Ran's "A Private Life". *PORTAL Journal of Multidisciplinary International Studies, 3*(2), 1–20.

Shi-xu. (2014). *Chinese discourse studies*. Hampshire, UK: Palgrave Macmillan.

Shi-xu. (2015). Towards a cultural methodology of human communication research: A Chinese example. In L. Tsung, & W. Wang (Eds.), *Contemporary Chinese discourse and social practice in China* (pp. 45–58). Amsterdam: John Benjamins.

Stout, P. A., Villegas, J., & Jennings, N. A. (2004). Images of mental illness in the media: Identifying gaps in the research. *Schizophrenia Bulletin, 30*(3), 543–561.

Tang, L., & Bie, B. (2015). Narratives about mental illnesses in China: The voices of Generation Y. *Health Communication, 31*(2), 171–181.

Thornicroft, A., Goulden, R., Shefer, G., Rhydderch, D., Rose, D., Williams, P., Thornicroft, G., & Henderson, C. (2013). Newspaper coverage of mental illness in England 2008–2011. *British Journal of Psychiatry, 202*(55), s64–s69.

Tian, H. (2012). Discursive production of teaching quality assessment report: A Critical Discourse Analysis. In P. Chilton, H. Tian, & R. Wodak (Eds.), *Discourse and socio-political transformations in contemporary China* (pp. 85–104). Amsterdam: John Benjamins.

Tian, H. (2015). Discourse and public sphere in China: A study of the Wu Ying lawsuit case. In L. Tsung, & W. Wang (Eds.), *Contemporary Chinese discourse and social practice in China* (pp. 27–44). Amsterdam: John Benjamins.

Traphagan. J. W. (2000). *Taming oblivion: Aging bodies and the fear of senility in Japan*. New York: State University of New York Press.

Tseng, W. (1986). Chinese psychiatry: Development and characteristics. In J. L. Cox (Ed.), *Transcultural psychiatry* (pp. 274–290). London: Crown Helm.

van Dijk, T. A. (1988a). *News analysis: Case studies of international and national news in the press*. Hillsdale, N.J: Lawrence Erlbaum.

van Dijk, T. A. (1988b). *News as discourse*. Hillsdale, N.J: Lawrence Erlbaum.

van Dijk, T. A. (2000). *Ideology: A multidisciplinary approach*. Thousand Oaks, CA: SAGE.

van Dijk, T. A. (2009). Critical Discourse Studies: A sociocognitive approach. In R. Wodak, & M. Meyer (Eds.), *Methods of critical discourse analysis* (pp. 62–86). London: SAGE.

van Dijk, T. A. (2014). Discourse, cognition, society. In J. Angermuller, D. Maingueneau, & R. Wodak (Eds.), *Discourse Studies reader: Main currents in theory and analysis* (pp. 388–399). Amsterdam: John Benjamins.

van Dijk, T. A. (2015). Critical Discourse Analysis. In D. Tannen, H. E. Hamilton, & D. Schiffrin (Eds.), *The handbook of discourse analysis* (pp. 466–485). Malden, MA: Wiley Blackwell.

van Dorn, R., Volavka, J., & Johnson, N. (2012). Mental disorder and violence: Is there a relationship beyond substance use? *Social Psychiatry and Psychiatric Epidemiology, 47*(3), 487–503.

van Leeuwen, T. (2007). Legitimation in discourse and communication. *Discourse and Communication, 1*(1), 91–112.

van Leeuwen, T. (2009). Discourse as the recontextualization of social practice: A guide. In R. Wodak, & M. Meyer (Eds.), *Methods of critical discourse analysis* (pp. 144–161). London: SAGE.

Varshney, M., Mahapatra, A., Krishnan, V., Gupta, R., & Deb, K. S. (2016). Violence and mental illness: What is the true story? *Journal of Epidemiology and Community Health, 70*(3), 223–225.

Wahl, O. (2003). News media portrayal of mental illness: Implications for public policy. *American Behavioral Scientist, 46*(12), 1594–1600.

Wahl, O., Wood, A., & Richards, R. (2002). Newspaper coverage of mental illness: Is it changing? *Psychiatric Rehabilitation Skills, 6*(1), 9–31.

Wang, W. (2015). Co-construction of migrant workers' identities on a TV talk show in China. In L. Tsung, & W. Wang (Ed.), *Contemporary Chinese discourse and social practice in China* (pp. 125–142). Amsterdam: John Benjamins.

Wang, W., & Tsung, L. (2015). Contemporary Chinese discourse from sociolinguistic perspectives. In L. Tsung, & W. Wang (Eds.), *Contemporary Chinese discourse and social practice in China* (pp. 1–10). Amsterdam: John Benjamins.

Wang, X. (2011). From asylum to museum: The discourse of insanity and schizophrenia in Shen Congwen's 1949 transition. *Modern Chinese Literature and Culture, 23*(1), 133–168.

Whitley, R., Adeponle, A., & Miller, A. R. (2015). Comparing gendered and generic representations of mental illness in Canadian newspapers: An exploration of the chivalry hypothesis. *Social Psychiatry and Psychiatric Epidemiology, 50*(2), 325–333.

Whitley, R., & Berry, S. (2013). Trends in newspaper coverage of mental illness in Canada: 2005–2010. *Canadian Journal of Psychiatry, 58*(2), 107–112.

Whitley, R., & Wang, J. W. (2017). Good news? A longitudinal analysis of newspaper portrayals of mental illness in Canada 2005 to 2015. *Canadian Journal of Psychiatry, 62*(4), 278–285.

Wodak, R. (1996). *Disorders of discourse*. London: Longman.

Wodak, R. (2014). The discourse of exclusion: Xenophobia, racism and anti-Semitism. In J. Angermuller, D. Maingueneau, & R. Wodak (Eds.), *Discourse Studies reader: Main currents in theory and analysis* (pp. 400–410). Amsterdam: John Benjamins.

Wodak, R., & Meyer, M. (2009). Critical Discourse Analysis: History, agenda, theory and methodology. In R. Wodak, & M. Meyer (Eds.), *Methods of critical discourse analysis* (pp. 1–33). London: SAGE.

Wu, H. Y. J., & Cheng, A. T. A. (2017). A history of mental healthcare in Taiwan. In H. Minas, & M. Lewis (Eds.), *Mental health in Asia and the Pacific: Historical and cultural perspectives* (pp. 107–121). Boston, MA: Springer.

Xia, Z., & Zhang, M. (1981). History and present status of modern psychiatry in China. *Chinese Medical Journal, 94*(5), 277–282.

Yang, X. (2011). Configuring female sickness and recovery: Chen Ran and Anni Baobei. *Modern Chinese Literature and Culture, 23*(1), 169–196.

Yang, Y., & Parrott, S. (2018). Schizophrenia in Chinese and U.S. online news media: Exploring cultural influence on the mediated portrayal of schizophrenia. *Health Communication, 33*(5), 553–561.

Yip, K. S. (2007). *Mental health service in the People's Republic of China: Current status and future developments.* New York: Nova Science Publishers.

You, Z., Chen, J., & Hong, Z. (2012). Discursive construction of Chinese foreign policy: A diachronic analysis of the Chinese government's *Annual Work Report* to the NPC. In P. Chilton, H. Tian, & R. Wodak (Eds.), *Discourse and socio-political transformations in contemporary China* (pp. 105–126). Amsterdam: John Benjamins.

Zhang, Q. (2012). The discursive construction of the social stratification order in reforming China. In P. Chilton, H. Tian, & R. Wodak (Eds.), *Discourse and socio-political transformations in contemporary China* (pp. 19–38). Amsterdam: John Benjamins.

Zhang, Y., Jin, Y., & Tang, Y. (2015). Framing depression: Cultural and organizational influences on coverage of a public health threat and attribution of responsibilities in Chinese news media, 2000–2012. *Journalism and Mass Communication Quarterly, 92*(1), 99–120.

Zhuang, X. Y., Wong, D. F. K., Cheng, C. W., & Pan, S. M. (2017). Mental health literacy, stigma and perception of causation of mental illness among Chinese people in Taiwan. *International Journal of Social Psychiatry, 63*(6), 498–507.

2 Comparative settings, newspapers, reports, and themes

This book examines how contemporary Chinese-language print news media texts from mainland China, Hong Kong, and Taiwan discursively construct severe mental illness. All three geographical locations are culturally Chinese, yet they have distinct social and political histories. My previous work shows that this can impact how Chinese-language texts from these important Chinese societies construct mental illness and related disorders (Ramsay 2008, 2013, 2016).

Approaches to and management of severe mental illness in greater China over the ages

In explicating the construction of severe mental illness in contemporary Chinese-language print media text from the three geographical locations, it is important to be aware of the social significance of severe mental illness in Chinese culture over time (Gallois & Callan 1997; Schiffrin 1994; Shi-xu 2014, 2015). Severe mental illness in China was characterised as early as the Han dynasty (260 BCE to 220 AD). At the time, the ancient medical text *Yellow Emperor's Internal Canon* [皇帝内经], writes about psychotic illness, adopting the colloquial expression madness [狂] (Chiu 1986; Hsueh-Shih 1995; Ng 1990; Tseng 1973a). Analogous mention of depressive illness, however, appears much later during the Ming dynasty (1368–1644). This is because such illness was generally somatised during the imperial era (Kleinman 1986). Bodily symptoms of depression, in fact, continued to be the dominant expression until quite recent times (Kleinman 1986; Lin 1985).

The prevailing attitudes towards and beliefs about severe mental illness in imperial China (pre-1912) were heavily shaped by Confucian teachings. These teachings emphasised the importance of maintaining social hierarchy, social order, social stability, and social contribution. People with a severe mental illness, most notably psychotic illness, publicly violated these key social tenets, through their disruptive behaviour and inability to productively contribute to the well-being of their families and the progress and development of the communities in which they lived (Baum 2018; Pearson 1996; Traphagan 2000). This, together with their apparent absence of valued human traits such as "commiseration," "shame," "humility," and "moral judgment" (Tseng 1973b, p. 193), degraded their personhood to the extent that they were no longer worthy of everyday society. As a result, they were burdens and embarrassments to their families (Baum 2018; Traphagan 2000), who were left with no alternative but to forcibly confine them at home or end their lives (Baum 2018; Chiu 1981). In addition, the genetic taint that accompanied severe mental illness, which is comprehensively discussed in Dikötter's (1998) book (see the Chapter 1 section on Chinese discourse studies on mental illness), added to a family's loss of face, due to the Confucian emphasis on patrilineal continuity. By late imperial times, the state had made families of people with a severe mental illness legally bound "to report the existence of an insane family member and keep him [sic] in strict confinement" (Chiu 1981, p. 81). Baum (2018, p. 79) cites Beijing municipal legislation from the early twentieth century, which tellingly declares that " '[t]hose who negligently allow lunatics, rabid dogs, or other dangerous animals to roam the streets or enter other peoples' houses' could be detained for up to fifteen days and fined up to fifteen yuan."

The systematic institutionalisation of those with a severe mental illness in designated psychiatric asylums became more common in the early twentieth century (Baum 2018). Western missionaries played a significant role in this (Chou 2006; Hsueh-Shih 1995; Kleinman 1986; Pearson 1996; Ran, Xiang, Simpson et al. 2005; Tseng 1986). China had become a republic in 1912, a time when eugenic thinking was gaining currency. The state, therefore, became aware of the need to remove these deemed damaged individuals from everyday society and place them in institutional care. At the same time, the state explicitly regulated their reproductive rights (Dikötter 1998). The popularisation of eugenic thought amongst the elites and the cultural status of those with a severe mental illness as non-persons ensured little public resistance to the legislative restrictions placed on their reproductive rights. Such restrictions continue through to the present day in mainland China.

The Western practice of psychiatry emerged during the Republican era, around the 1930s (Baum 2018; Hsueh-Shih 1995; Kleinman 1986; Pearson 1991). It was largely limited to urban centres where there were significant foreign enclaves (Baum 2018). The eugenic vision that also had entered from the West was embraced by the Republican authorities and elites, in part, due to the very presence of these foreign enclaves (Baum 2018; Dikötter 1998). They symbolised the degraded state of China at the time, as the "sick man of the East" [东方病夫]. One way to restore China's health and status in the world would be to improve the quality of the population. This could be achieved by reducing the number of deemed imperfect or inferior people, which in prevailing cultural thinking included those with a severe mental illness (Baum 2018; Dikötter 1998). Most notably, if they were unable to reproduce, they would eventually be eliminated from society (Baum 2018).

Republican-era China was racked by the Japanese invasion and the Chinese Civil War throughout the late 1930s and the 1940s. Around this time, the Nationalist Party government began to enthusiastically embrace contemporary neuropsychiatry (Baum 2018). This brought about the recasting of "madness" as "mental illness" in official circles (Baum 2018, p. 111). Baum (2018) states that the Nationalist Party government did so in political self-interest, as neuropsychiatry embodied the

> intensely modernist characteristics of hygiene, bureaucratic rationalism, and scientific expertise – characteristics that could easily signal the Guomindang's [Nationalist Party's] distance from its warlord forerunners, and hence provide justification for its political mandate to rule.
>
> (p. 129)

National Party rule ended in 1949. Having triumphed, the Communists immediately set about building a new socialist China. The Soviet influence was strong in the early years of socialist reconstruction in the 1950s, including in the area of neuropsychiatry (Kleinman 1986; Pearson 1996; Ran, Xiang, Simpson et al. 2005; Tseng 1986; Xue, Shi, Knoll et al. 2015; Yan 1985). However, the treatment and care of those with a severe mental illness in the early Communist era held a low priority, at a time of spirited nation-building and sweeping land reform. Internal political jockeying characterised the early 1960s, erupting into the Cultural Revolution in 1966, a period of radical leftist ideological dominance that lasted for ten years. During this time, the authorities were highly sceptical of foreign ideas and influence, including those from the erstwhile Communist ally the Soviet Union. This impacted the state's official line on severe mental illness. It was deemed to be a product of, or manifestation of, incorrect political thinking (Baum 2018). Systematic, collective political re-education, therefore, would solve this problem, rather than neuropsychiatry that was focused on individual concerns and experience. It was unproblematic that this required the removal of those with a severe mental illness from everyday society, as such action aligned with prevailing stigmatic cultural attitudes and beliefs.

The collective correcting of people's political thinking would unlikely have cured their severe mental illness during the Cultural Revolution. There is scant documentation of what actually became of people with a severe mental illness during this decade of intense social and political upheaval. Literary works written after the Cultural Revolution paint a bleak picture of the torment and death of those with a severe mental illness, in particular psychotic illness, during this time (see previous chapter's section on Chinese discourse studies on mental illness). Anecdotal communication shared by mentally well people who lived through the Cultural Revolution broadly confirms the literary portrayal of severe mental illness, at least for those who suffered from the illness and lived, as most mainland Chinese did, in smaller towns and villages away from urban centres. A life on the margins in such locations also characterised the early years of the reform period that followed the Cultural Revolution, as I have witnessed first-hand. At this time, the deaths of people who manifestly suffered from a severe mental illness were barely noticed by a largely indifferent local community.

After Mao Zedong's death in 1976, Deng Xiaoping eventually seized power and implemented the Open Door reform program. Since the turn of the twenty-first century, there have been modest improvements in mental health care in mainland China (Ran, Xiang, Simpson et al. 2005; Xu, Li, Xu et al. 2017). Western biomedical approaches dominate contemporary practice. Although there has been no de-institutionalisation program as carried out in many Western countries, there are a number of well-equipped, soundly run psychiatric institutions (Phillips, Chen, Diesfeld et al. 2013; Xu, Li, Xu et al. 2017), such as those set up with the assistance of the charitable Richmond Fellowship of Hong Kong [利民會]. Despite modest advances, mainland China still lacks suitably qualified mental health professionals, particularly in rural and remote areas (Hu, Rohrbaugh, Deng et al. 2017; Liu & Page 2016; Patel, Xiao, Chen et al. 2016; Phillips, Chen, Diesfeld et al. 2013; Xu, Li, Xu et al. 2017). In 2015, the World Health Organization recorded 1.49 psychiatrists practicing in mainland China per 100,000 population (Mendelson & Lin 2016). The comparable figure for Australia in 2011 was 12.76 psychiatrists per 100,000 population (Mendelson & Lin 2016). Prevalence rates of severe mental illness in both settings are broadly similar. At present, the mainland Chinese government is implementing a five-year Mental Health Plan (2015–2020) that seeks to substantially increase the number of qualified mental health professionals nationwide, albeit to a level still far below that of Australia (Hu, Rohrbaugh, Deng et al. 2017).

Social stigma against severe mental illness remains a big problem in present-day mainland China (Patel, Xiao, Chen et al. 2016; Xu, Li, Xu et al. 2017). This stems from the long-standing negative attitudes towards and beliefs about severe mental illness in culturally Chinese communities. The previous chapter outlines how these attitudes and beliefs are borne out in contemporary texts from a number of genres. This book, of course, explores this phenomenon in contemporary news texts. The enduring intense stigma is a contributory factor to the low contact rate with formal mental health services in mainland China. Most people with a severe mental illness in mainland China have never accessed such services (Liu 2008; Liu & Page 2016; Mendelson & Lin 2016). Numbers have barely improved over decades, despite the many advances in the provision of mental healthcare. Since the vast majority of those with a severe mental illness in mainland China live at home with their families (Fan & Wang 2015; Ran, Xiang, Simpson et al. 2005), the burden that they place on them is immense. Mendelson and Lin (2016, p. 766) tellingly point out that, in 2011, "the poverty rate of the families of patients with mental health disorders was 20 times higher than [mainland] China's average family poverty rate." In addition, families are legally culpable for any socially disruptive behaviour and actions of a family member with a severe mental illness (Every-Palmer, Brink, Chern et al. 2014; Phillips, Chen, Diesfeld et al. 2013; Topiwala, Wang, & Fazel 2012). As noted earlier in this section, such prescription of familial accountability dates back to imperial times (Chiu 1981).

In 2013, the national government enacted the *Mental Health Law of the People's Republic of China* [中华人民共和国精神卫生法] (Li, Gutheil, & Hu 2016; Patel, Xiao, Chen et al. 2016; Xue, Shi, Knoll et al. 2015). This act, for the first time since the Communist victory in 1949, formalised the rights of citizens with a severe mental illness and the responsibilities of their mental health professionals (Fan & Wang 2015; Mendelson & Lin 2016; Phillips, Chen, Diesfeld et al. 2013). The act is comprehensively modelled, like comparable Western mental health legislation, on World Health Organization best practices (Fan & Wang 2015; Mendelson & Lin 2016). Mendelson and Lin (2016) point to its "procedural protection against improper involuntary [hospital] admission and treatment" (p. 775). Deliberate malicious abuse of mental health admission and treatment practices against mentally well citizens had become legendary, such that it was colloquially coined as *bei jingshenbing* [被精神病], roughly translating as to be made a mentally ill person (Mendelson & Lin 2016). Mendelson and Lin (2016) and Phillips, Chen, Diesfeld et al. (2013), however, note the absence of access to independent judicial reviews of health professional decisions, of the kinds that provide checks and balances in Western countries such as Australia. Fan and Wang (2015) add that many health professionals simply ignore the new mental health act, especially in rural and remote regions. Others, meanwhile, use it strategically for their own benefit, or apply it fastidiously to the detriment of those with a severe mental illness (Fan & Wang 2015).

The approaches to and management of severe mental illness in Hong Kong contrast with those in mainland China and Taiwan, due to its relatively unbroken history of provision of health and social work services by both government and charitable organisations (Jones 1990; Yip 1998). Similar to the Western historical trend, approaches to and management of severe mental illness in Hong Kong have evolved from a primarily custodial paradigm, through pharmacotherapy to a contemporary community-based rehabilitative paradigm that is heavily informed by client-centred social work theory (Mak 1991; Yip 1998). This is unsurprising given that, for most of the period in question, Hong Kong was a colony of Great Britain. The territory only shed its colonial status and became integrated into the People's Republic of China as a Special Administrative Region [香港特別行政区] in 1997.

One of the first semi-charitable bodies to care for people with a severe mental illness in Hong Kong in the early colonial period was Tung Wah Hospital [東華醫院]. It was "the first general hospital for Chinese in Hong Kong," being established in the late nineteenth century, and is still active today (Yip 1998, p. 47). During this period, non-Chinese people with a severe mental illness were repatriated by the colonial authorities to their home countries (Yip 1998). Custodial care in psychiatric asylums became the leading approach in colonial Hong Kong during the early twentieth century and leading up to World War Two (Mak 1991; Yip 1998). This was also the case on the mainland and in colonial Taiwan. At the time, many Chinese people with a severe mental illness in Hong Kong were even expatriated to a psychiatric asylum in Guangzhou on the mainland (Yip 1998). From 1912 to 1949, mainland China was officially under Nationalist Party rule and still an ally of Great Britain. Such practices ceased after the Communist victory on the mainland in 1949 (Yip 1998).

Throughout the 1950s and 1960s, fledgling mental health advocacy groups emerged in Hong Kong, together with the ascendancy of pharmacotherapy in the approach to and management of severe mental illness (Mak 1991; Yip 1998). Closely following this came community-based rehabilitative services, "in the form of sheltered workshops, half-way houses, rehabilitation farms and psychiatric units in general hospitals" (Yip 1998, p. 49. See also Mak 1991). These services were delivered by both government and charitable bodies. They continued to expand throughout the 1970s and 1980s (Mak 1991). By the 1990s, the central role of social workers in the multidisciplinary, rehabilitative, community care of people with a severe mental illness became clearly recognised (Yip 1998). This enabled great progress in the area, under the tutelage of academic pioneers such as Professor Veronica Pearson at the University of Hong Kong, as well as local charitable bodies such as the aforementioned Richmond Fellowship of Hong Kong. As a consequence, some facets of present-day approaches to and management of severe mental illness are distinct from those in neighbouring mainland China and Taiwan. This stems from a greater emphasis that is placed on nurturing the independent living skills, quality of life, and employment of people with severe mental illness in Hong Kong (Hung 2008).

Nonetheless, ongoing local resistance to the de-institutionalisation of people with a severe mental illness, which is largely informed by the long-standing Chinese cultural stigma, contributes to an enduring presence in Hong Kong, as on the mainland and in Taiwan, of long-term residential psychiatric institutions that are located far away from everyday society (Mak 1991; Yip 1998). The most well known of these institutions in Hong Kong is Castle Peak Hospital [青山醫院] (Mak 1991). In local Cantonese, the expression "Castle Peak" (*lit.* Green Mountain) [青山] metonymically denotes, in a derogatory way, "madhouse" or "nutcase." Cultural stigma may also contribute to the relatively low number of psychiatrists in Hong Kong, although their numbers are steadily increasing over time (Heifetz 2016; World Health Organization 2011). There currently are five psychiatrists per 100,000 population in Hong Kong, which is just under half of the number in Australia and three times the number in mainland China (Heifetz 2016).

The approaches to and management of severe mental illness in Taiwan, like those in mainland China, have been impacted by major social and political upheaval and vicissitudes. Japanese colonial rule during most of the first half of the twentieth century treated local people as subjects lay open to the scientific gaze of the curious occupier (Chou 2006; Wu & Cheng 2017). This included those with a severe mental illness. The colonial authorities opened

Taiwan's first psychiatric asylum in 1922 (Chou 2006). It was patterned on similar institutions in Japan, which, in turn, had been modelled on European psychiatric asylums (Chou 2006). After the Japanese departure on their defeat in World War Two and the subsequent Communist victory on the mainland in 1949, the Nationalist Party ruled over Taiwan as an authoritative dictatorship until the late 1980s. During this time, the government's approach to mental health and its management largely carried on practices from the Republican era on the mainland (Chou 2006). Elements of modern psychiatry emerged on Taiwan, but with most of the government attention directed towards short-term institutional care for people with a severe mental illness, passing most responsibility to their families (Chou 2006; Wu & Cheng 2017). Overall, mental healthcare remained a low priority for the Nationalist Party government during the greater part of the dictatorship (Chou 2006; Wu & Cheng 2017).

Since democratisation, there have been notable advances in mental healthcare in Taiwan, in particular in community-based mental health services and treatment (Chou 2006; Wu 2008; Wu & Cheng 2017). These advances in many ways mirror those pursued on the mainland and in Hong Kong. Impressively, the relative number of qualified mental health professionals in present-day Taiwan is on a par with that for Australia (Lu, Tung, & Ely 2016). Since the 1990s, people in Taiwan have also had ready access to a well-equipped public health system (Chou 2006; Wu 2008), with the exception of those living in the remote areas (Lu, Tung, & Ely 2016). Yet, paradoxically, at the same time, a large-scale, gated, residential facility continues to permanently house several hundred people with severe mental illness in the well-known Hall of Dragon Metamorphoses [龍發堂]. This religious institution has operated, albeit with occasional controversy, in southern Taiwan since the 1970s (Chou 2006; Wu & Cheng 2017). In 2018, the future of the facility, once again, was being called into question. The residents of the Hall of Dragon Metamorphoses follow Buddhist folk teachings and religious practices, living a cloistered existence that is free of pharmacotherapy and, in line with long-standing stigmatic attitudes and beliefs in culturally Chinese communities, removed from everyday society. Locally, the name of this facility has metonymically denoted "madhouse" or "nutcase," in a similar derogatory way to the expression "Castle Peak" in Hong Kong. The names of some local psychiatric institutions in mainland China also are used in this metonymical, derogatory way, such as the Daizhuang [岱庄] facility in Shandong province.

In 1990, the Taiwan government enacted a Mental Health Law that is deemed progressive but also paternalistic, by world standards (Chou 2006; Wu & Cheng 2017). The act upholds the traditionally central role of the Chinese family in severe mental illness, legalistically codifying it in the expression "*Baohuren* (保護人, *Tutelar*)" or "guardian" (Chou 2006, p. 14). This places Taiwanese families in a position of legal responsibility that is akin to that faced by their mainland counterparts. In recent decades, non-governmental charitable trusts like the John Tung Foundation [財團法人董氏基金會] have invested significantly in community psychoeducation, especially targeting depression in young people (Ramsay 2008; Wu & Cheng 2017). Wu and Cheng (2017), however, observe that offsetting positive investment of this kind is the ongoing problematic reporting of mental health matters by the news media in Taiwan.

Severe mental illness in present-day greater China

While lay attitudes towards and beliefs about severe mental illness broadly align across greater China, progress in the delivery of mental healthcare varies across geographical locations. Following the implementation of the post-Mao Open Door reforms from 1978 onward, mainland China has made great progress in addressing the negative legacies of the Cultural Revolution, namely, poor public understanding about mental illness; an underdeveloped mental health service infrastructure; and a lack of adequately trained personnel. There, however, has been much slower improvement in public understanding about severe mental illness (Patel, Xiao, Chen et al. 2016; Pearson 1992, 1996; Ran, Xiang, Simpson et al. 2005; Xu, Li, Xu et al. 2017). A long-standing intense cultural stigma against severe mental illness continues to shape widely held attitudes and beliefs across mainland China (Guo 2016; Kleinman, Yan, Jun et al. 2011; Ramsay 2013; Xu, Li, Xu et al. 2017). These entrenched stigmatic attitudes and beliefs cast people with a severe mental illness as "dangerous," "dysfunctional," "incompetent," and "weak" (Wang & Liu 2016, p. 357). Zhang, Jin, and Tang (2015, p. 100) note that the "low levels of mental health literacy across Chinese society have also contributed to negative public attitudes and lack of support in health policies, including mental illness prevention and health care access and parity." This impacts the tens of millions of citizens who suffer from depression and the several million citizens who suffer from schizophrenia in mainland China today (Chan, Zhao, Meng et al. 2015; Zhang, Jin, & Tang 2015). Zhang, Jin, and Tang (2015, p. 100) tellingly predict that these existing challenges will only escalate in the future, with mental illness likely to "become the largest burden on public health in China by 2020," based on World Health Organization projections. This requires urgent attention, given mainland China's huge population, currently numbering around 1.4 billion people.

Since its integration with the People's Republic of China in 1997, Hong Kong has continued to develop "a relatively coherent and proactive approach" to social policy in Hong Kong, which currently advances "liberal notions of client-centredness and client-empowerment" (Ramsay 2016, p. 67). The population of Hong Kong currently numbers more than seven million. Ho, Potash, Fong et al. (2015) claim that 24% of this population suffer from a mental illness, a smaller percentage of whom suffer from severe forms, the focus of this book. Yet, offsetting Hong Kong's relatively enlightened social policy towards mental illness, social stigma remains intense and widespread, as it does across the Chinese diaspora (Ho, Potash, Fong et al. 2015; Mann & Chong 2016;

Rosenberg 2018). Ho, Potash, Fong et al. (2015, p. 199) revealingly point out that only a very small percentage of people with a mental illness in Hong Kong are "currently receiving psychiatric services." They attribute this low percentage to the prevailing social stigma, amongst other factors.

Across the strait, present-day democratic Taiwan has a population of more than twenty-three million people. Chen, Yip, Tsai et al. (2012) describe the region "[a]s a newly industrialized country that models the Western style of living, enjoys media freedom, and yet is also deeply rooted in its Chinese cultural heritage" (p. 144). As such, it remains culturally Chinese. This occurs despite its locally well celebrated, yet low in overall number, indigenous populations; and its visibly active, yet low in overall number, Christian communities (Kuo 2008; Lo 2011; Ramsay 2016). Accordingly, people's views on mental illness in Taiwan are strongly shaped by long-standing Chinese cultural norms, values, and scripts that impact on those with a mental illness in highly stigmatic ways (Han, Lin, Liao et al. 2015; Mellor, Carne, Shen et al. 2013; Zhuang, Wong, Cheng et al. 2017). Fu, Lee, Gunnell et al. (2013) estimate that around 24% of the people in Taiwan suffer from a mental illness, which very closely aligns with the figure for Hong Kong. Zhuang, Wong, Cheng et al. (2017) cite a similar figure, while noting a very high prevalence rate for elderly people in Taiwan. A smaller percentage of people suffer from severe mental illness, which is the focus of this book.

The Chinese-language newspapers

This book analyses recent reports in three leading Chinese-language broadsheet newspapers from mainland China, Hong Kong, and Taiwan, namely, the *People's Daily* [人民日报], *Ming Pao* [明報], and *Liberty Times* [自由時報], respectively. These newspapers are chosen due to their mainstream status, wide circulations, and local ownership and production. The *People's Daily* is a mainland Chinese national daily newspaper that acts as an official messenger for the Chinese Communist Party and the mainland Chinese government (Brady 2002; Cao 2014; Lee 2015; Yang & Parrott 2018). It "set[s] the tone" for reporting by the numerous regional and sectional newspapers that currently operate across mainland China (Sandby-Thomas 2014, p. 53). This regulatory role, its official status, and its continuing high circulation figures make it one of the most influential newspapers in mainland China today and, so, a prime choice for analysis in this book (Peng & Tang 2010; Sandby-Thomas 2014). The newspaper is published in a broadsheet format, with a daily circulation figure of around 2.5 million (BBC News 2013). At present, there are approximately two thousand newspapers operating across mainland China (Lee 2015). Most of them are smaller "populist" and "non-Party" commercial ventures (Tong 2014, p. 138). The party and state, nevertheless, closely monitor, and sometimes censor, them (Brady 2009; Lee 2015; Shephard 2017). This is done under the auspices of a Central Propaganda Department, whose "primary function is to mobilise public opinion behind party policies" (Lee 2015, p. 120). If any newspapers happen to report on sensitive political or social topics in ways that contravene these policies, they face punitive sanctions and bans, staff imprisonment, or newspaper closure (Brady 2002, 2009; Lee 2015). Severe mental illness is one such topic that the party and state designate as sensitive. This is because it is potentially problematic for a mainland Chinese government that politically prioritises social harmony and social stability [维和维稳] (Brady 2009; Cao 2014; Choy 2016; Sandby-Thomas 2014).

Ming Pao is a leading commercial daily newspaper in Hong Kong. *BBC Monitoring* (2016, n.p.) describes it as "a well-respected, independent Hong Kong daily" that "top[ped] the list of the most credible newspapers" in a "survey of public evaluation on media credibility conducted by the Centre for Communication and Public Opinion Survey of the Chinese University of Hong Kong." The newspaper is published in a broadsheet format, with a current daily circulation figure of 140,000, according to Factiva. It is chosen for analysis in this book due to its relatively high circulation figures, media eminence, and middle-of-the-road political stance. Other high-circulation Chinese-language newspapers in Hong Kong, such as *Oriental Daily News* [東方日報], *Apple Daily* [蘋果日報], and *Headline Daily* [頭條日報], are renowned for their tabloid sensationalism, and, in the case of *Apple Daily*, its transparent political stance against the national government of the People's Republic of China in Beijing.

Liberty Times is a leading commercial daily newspaper in Taiwan. Chen (2011) states that it takes a more liberal stance in its reporting of social and political issues, with a readership of "mainly Taiwanese people who support Taiwan's independence and are concerned about sovereignty" (p. 699). This contrasts with the competing, but less commercially successful, *United Daily News* [聯合報] and *China Times* [中國時報], whose political stances tend to be more favourable towards the government of the People's Republic of China in Beijing; and whose political stances plainly support a One-China policy, namely, that the regions making up greater China, which, of course, include Taiwan, form a single sovereign entity, that is, "China." No prominent newspapers in Taiwan take a purely middle-of-the-road political stance. *Liberty Times* is published in a broadsheet format, with a current daily circulation figure of 626,392, according to Factiva. This is the highest figure for all newspapers in Taiwan. Its closest commercial competitor, *Apple Daily* (Taiwan) [蘋果日報], is Hong Kong owned and has a proclivity for tabloid sensationalism. As such, *Liberty Times* is chosen for analysis in this book, due to its high circulation figures, wholly local ownership and production, and more measured broadsheet reporting.

The news reports

The Factiva keyword search found a total of 205 news reports that make mention of severe mental illness in their headlines and lead paragraphs, or in the main event of a report in the absence of a lead paragraph. These schematic components of a news text represent the uppermost levels of its superstructural hierarchy (van Dijk 1988a, 2015). All of the news reports were retained for analysis, regardless of the extent to which they deal with severe mental illness. This is in line with the assertion by Wahl, Wood, and Richards (2002) that any mention of mental illness in a news report, at least in the uppermost levels of its superstructural hierarchy, is discursively significant. The analysis in Chapters 3, 4, and 5 confirm that the number of sourced news reports is sufficient to reach saturation level, whereby definitive trends are clearly evident across the newspaper corpora (Corbin & Strauss 2008). Appendices 1, 2, and 3 list the following details for each of the 205 news reports:

- assigned reference number [#1-#205], to aid identification throughout this book.
- the Chinese-language headline.
- "faithful" English-language translation of its headline.
- section of the newspaper where it is published.
- the date of publication.
- total word count, in number of Chinese characters.
- name of the mental illness it reports on.
- broad thematic category it belongs to, for example, medical report or crime report. The topical focus of a majority of the sentences in a report determine its thematic category (Paterson 2007).

This information can be readily used to find the entire news report on the internet. As stated in the Chapter 1 section on the analysis of Chinese-language print media reports on severe mental illness, this book analyses the entirety of every news report.

The Factiva keyword search covered a six-month time period from mid-December 2015 to mid-June 2016 for all three newspapers. For the *People's Daily*, an additional search covering the preceding six-month period (mid-June 2015 to mid-December 2015) was carried out, due to the comparatively low number of reports obtained for the period covering mid-December 2015 to mid-June 2016. This was undertaken to ascertain whether the numerical and discursive characteristics of the *People's Daily* news reports from the six-month period common to all three newspapers are replicated over a longer period of time and in a larger corpus.

The comparatively low number of *People's Daily* reports obtained for the six-month period common to all three newspapers likely is because severe mental illness is a politically sensitive topic for the mainland Chinese authorities, for whom social harmony and social stability are of paramount concern (Brady 2009; Cao 2014; Choy 2016; Sandby-Thomas 2014). As a result, they would seek to "restrict" and "manag[e]" visible reporting on it, as they do with other "politically sensitive health-related issues [...] such as SARS, AIDS, and drug addiction" (Brady 2008, p. 29). Peng and Tang (2010, p. 703) conversely detect "significant coverage" of mental illness in mainland Chinese newspapers, when compared to their counterparts in the United States. They, however, do not name the specific mental illnesses that are reported on in their wider study of health coverage in mainland Chinese newspapers. They may have been milder forms of mental illness. Nor do they compare the level of coverage in mainland Chinese newspapers with that in counterparts from across greater China. Yang and Parrott (2018) further find that mainland Chinese online news media regularly report on schizophrenia, and do so more often than their counterparts in the United States. They, however, include reports that name the illness at any level of the news text superstructural hierarchy, although later excluding those that use the expression metaphorically. They, too, do not compare the level of coverage in mainland Chinese online news media with that in their counterparts from across greater China.

The Factiva keyword search for the six-month period common to all three newspapers matched seventeen *People's Daily* news reports on severe mental illness. An analogous Factiva search for the preceding six-month period covering mid-June 2015 to mid-December 2015 matched sixteen news reports, an almost identical number to the original six-month period. Figure 2.1 shows that the number of published news reports varies from month to month. September 2015 has the highest number, with six reports on unrelated events. March 2016 and August, October, November, and December 2015 each have only one or no report.

The seventeen *People's Daily* reports for the six-month period common to all three newspapers can be grouped into six broad thematic categories, based on their content, namely:

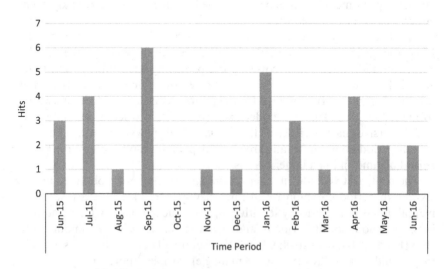

Figure 2.1 People's Daily keyword search matches ("hits"): mid-June 2015 to mid-June 2016.

1. current medical findings about severe mental illness and related disorders, such as prevalence rates, causes, early warning signs, and treatments, as well as available support services and public health measures.
2. government policy on severe mental illness.
3. celebrity experiences of severe mental illness.
4. crime and civil law where severe mental illness is implicated.
5. suicide where severe mental illness is at issue.
6. education and student mental health.

Appendix 1 shows that there are five medical reports, accounting for 29% of the corpus; four policy reports and four celebrity reports (24% each); two crime reports (12%); one suicide report (6%); and one education report (6%). Eight news reports (47%) deal directly or indirectly with generic severe mental illness [精神病], with the same number (47%) reporting on depression [抑郁症]. Only one report (6%) deals with schizophrenia, denoted by the conventional diagnostic label *jingshenfenlie* [精神分裂]. None report on psychosis [精神錯亂]. The appendix shows that five reports (29%) from this six-month period appear in the medical news section of the newspaper, with another four reports (24%) appearing in its entertainment news section. This reflects the higher proportion of medical reports and celebrity reports. Two reports (12%) each appear in the national news section and as opinion pieces, while one report (6%) each appears in the international, legal, culinary, and United Front news sections.[1] Most reporting on severe mental illness, therefore, appears as ancillary specialist news, rather than primary national news. Appendix 1 also shows that the length of the news reports from this six-month period range from 215 Chinese characters (approximately 160 English words) to 2,492 characters (approximately 1,870 English words), with an average of 991 characters (approximately 740 English words).

The sixteen *People's Daily* reports for the additional six-month period from mid-June 2015 to mid-December 2015 can similarly be grouped into six broad thematic categories, based on their content, namely:

1. current medical findings about severe mental illness and related disorders, such as prevalence rates, causes, early warning signs, and treatments, as well as available support services and public health measures.
2. government policy on severe mental illness.
3. celebrity experiences of severe mental illness.
4. suicide where severe mental illness is at issue.
5. crime where severe mental illness is implicated.
6. art history and severe mental illness.

The thematic categories for the *People's Daily* reports for both of the six-month time periods, therefore, closely align, except for art history supplanting education. These two outlying categories, nevertheless, only account for one news report each. Appendix 1 shows that other characteristics of the reports from the original six-month period also are replicated in the six-month period that precedes it. The preceding period only has only one more medical report and suicide report, two fewer celebrity reports, and one fewer crime report. It also has only one more report on generic severe mental illness [精神病] and schizophrenia, denoted by the conventional diagnostic label *jingshenfenlie* [精神分裂]; one fewer report on depression [抑郁症]; and, equally, no reports on psychosis [精神錯亂]. Once again, most of the reporting on severe mental illness appears as ancillary specialist news rather than primary national news. The appendix also shows that the length of the *People's Daily* reports from this six-month period range from 149 Chinese characters (approximately 110 English words) to 2,119 characters (approximately 1,590 English words), with an average of 890 characters (approximately 670 English words). This average broadly aligns with that of the original six-month period common to all three newspapers. Since the total number of *People's Daily* reports for each six-month period is almost identical, their total character counts also broadly align. What is more, when these two totals are summed together, the resulting character count approaches that of the *Ming Pao* and *Liberty Times* corpora.

The Factiva keyword search matched sixty-four *Ming Pao* news reports for the six-month period from mid-December 2015 to mid-June 2016. This figure is much higher than that for the *People's Daily* and more than sufficient to reach saturation level, whereby definitive trends are clearly evident across the newspaper corpora (Corbin & Strauss 2008). Figure 2.2 shows that there are around ten or so matches for each month, remembering that December and June are not full-month searches. The exception is March with fifteen reports.

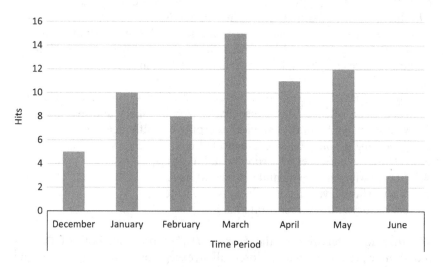

Figure 2.2 Ming Pao keyword search matches ("hits"): mid-December 2015 to mid-June 2016.

No single news event can explain this cluster of reports in March. The sixty-four *Ming Pao* reports can be grouped into six broad thematic categories, based on their content, namely:

1. crime where severe mental illness is implicated.
2. suicide where severe mental illness is at issue.
3. celebrity experiences of severe mental illness.
4. everyday personal experiences of severe mental illness.
5. current medical findings about severe mental illness, such as prevalence rates, causes, early warning signs, and treatments.
6. political issues and activism in severe mental illness.

All categories, bar the everyday personal experiences of severe mental illness, are common to the *People's Daily* reports, but in quite differing proportions. Appendix 2 shows that there are twenty-five crime reports (39%), nine suicide reports (14%), eight celebrity reports (13%), eight reports on the everyday personal experience (13%), seven medical reports (11%), and seven political reports (11%). Thirty-two reports (50%) deal directly or indirectly with generic severe mental illness [精神病]. Twenty-three reports (36%) deal with depression [抑鬱症], while twelve (19%) deal with schizophrenia, denoted both by the conventional diagnostic label *jingshenfenlie* [精神分裂], and the neutral neologism *sijueshitiao* [思覺失調]. One report (2%) deals with psychosis [精神錯亂]. Four reports deal with more than one of these illnesses. The appendix shows that thirty-seven (58%) of the reports appear in the newspaper's local Hong Kong news section. Another ten reports (16%) appear in special columns that print opinion pieces by experts, activists, people with a severe mental illness, and their family caregivers; seven reports (11%) appear in the entertainment news section; five reports (8%) appear in the mainland Chinese news section; four reports (6%) appear in the international news section; and one report (2%) appears in the education news section. Appendix 2 also shows that the length of the news reports range from 105 Chinese characters (approximately eighty English words) to 2,934 characters (approximately 2,200 English words), with an average of 619 characters (approximately 460 English words). Thus, on average, the *Ming Pao* reports are much shorter than their *People's Daily* counterparts.

The Factiva keyword search matched 108 *Liberty Times* news reports for the six-month period from mid-December 2015 to mid-June 2016. Figure 2.3 shows that there are around ten matches for most months, remembering that December and June are not full-month searches. January and March are clear exceptions, with double to triple the number of matches for the other months. No single news event contributes to these temporal clusters. An infamous random killing of a young girl on a Taipei street in late March 2016 only partially contributes, as the mental health status of the killer was not immediately ascertained. The reports can be grouped into eight broad thematic categories, based on their content, namely:

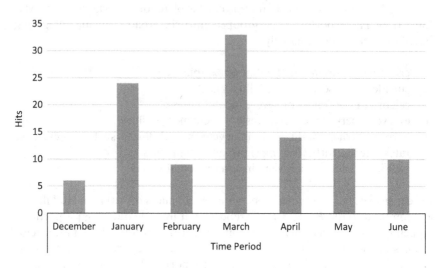

Figure 2.3 Liberty Times keyword search matches ("hits"): mid-December 2015 to mid-June 2016.

1. crime where severe mental illness is implicated.
2. celebrity experiences of severe mental illness.
3. current medical findings about severe mental illness, such as prevalence rates, causes, early warning signs and treatments, as well as available support services.
4. suicide where severe mental illness is at issue.
5. everyday personal experiences of severe mental illness.
6. political issues and activism in severe mental illness.
7. missing persons who have a severe mental illness.
8. finance and the psych-economy.

The first six categories are common to the *Ming Pao* reports. They also are common to the *People's Daily* reports, with the exception of the everyday personal experiences of severe mental illness. Appendix 3 shows that there are twenty-six crime reports, accounting for 24% of the *Liberty Times* corpus. There are twenty-one celebrity reports (19%); eighteen medical reports (17%); seventeen suicide reports (16%); twelve reports on the everyday personal experience (11%); and eleven political reports (10%). The additional two categories only have three reports in total, namely, two missing person reports (2%) and one finance report (1%). Seventeen news reports (16%) deal directly or indirectly with generic severe mental illness [精神病]. Eighty-three reports (77%) deal with depression [憂鬱症], while eight (7%) deal with schizophrenia, denoted both by the conventional diagnostic label *jingshenfenlie* [精神分裂], and the neutral neologism *sijueshitiao* [思覺失調].

No reports deal with psychosis [精神錯亂]. Thus, the *Liberty Times* reports deal with depression much more often than their *People's Daily* and *Ming Pao* counterparts do. The appendix shows that fifty-seven (53%) of the *Liberty Times* reports appear in the newspaper's local news section. This figure is very similar to that for the *Ming Pao* reports. Twenty reports (19%) appear in the entertainment news section, reflecting the high number of celebrity reports. Twelve reports (11%) appear in the medical news section; six (6%) appear in the lifestyle news; four (4%) appear in the finance news; with two (2%) each in the political news and international news sections. Only five reports (5%) appear in special columns that print opinion pieces and commentary by experts, activists, reporter-interviewers, and friends of people with a severe mental illness. Appendix 3 also shows that the length of the news reports ranges from 116 Chinese characters (approximately ninety English words) to 1,442 characters (approximately 1,080 English words), with an average of 425 characters (approximately 320 English words). Thus, while the *Liberty Times* reports well outnumber their *People's Daily* and *Ming Pao* counterparts, they tend to be much shorter in length, such that the total character count for each newspaper corpus is surprisingly similar. The *People's Daily* corpus, of course, covers a twelve-month, rather than a six-month, time period.

Comparative themes

The thematic categories are seemingly quite uniform across all three Chinese-language newspapers. Their reporting on severe mental illness consistently focuses on crime and social wrongdoing, such as sensational, ignominious suicide; the lives of celebrities and lay people; current medical issues and concerns; and political issues and activism. Paterson (2007) observed similar thematic patterning in U.K. newspaper reports on mental illness. The numerical predominance of thematic categories across the three Chinese-language newspapers, nevertheless, varies significantly. Crime where severe mental illness is implicated is the dominant theme in the Hong Kong and Taiwan newspapers, yet is one of the least common themes in the mainland Chinese newspaper. I call attention to the mainland Chinese authorities' current political emphasis on maintaining social harmony and social stability, in the previous section of this chapter. This political phenomenon may similarly account for the lower number of reports on crime where severe mental illness is implicated in the *People's Daily* when compared to *Ming Pao* and *Liberty Times*. This is because a key role of the party and state is to prevent crime. Reporting on crime at the levels found in *Ming Pao* and *Liberty Times* in mainland China's flagship national newspaper might suggest that the party and state have erred in their duty to properly take care of, manage, and control citizens who have a severe mental illness, and, accordingly, neglected their foremost political responsibility to maintain social harmony and social stability.

In Hong Kong and Taiwan, where the local press is not under the strict control of the governing authorities, reporting on crime where severe mental illness is implicated conversely dominates. This is especially so for *Ming Pao*, where 39% of reports deal with such crime. The corresponding figure for the second most common theme in the *Ming Pao* reports, namely, suicide where severe mental illness is at issue, is far lower, at just 14%. Although crime where severe mental illness is implicated is also the leading theme in the *Liberty Times* reports, it comprises a much lower overall percentage, at just 24%. While the *Liberty Times* reports deal with suicide where severe mental illness is at issue as often as their *Ming Pao* counterparts do, they report more on the lives of celebrities and current medical issues and concerns.

The thematic dominance of crime where severe mental illness is implicated in the reporting of *Ming Pao* and *Liberty Times* can be explained by its sensational value in these two commercial ventures (Angermeyer & Schulze 2001; Kesic, Ducat, & Thomas 2012). This appears to be especially so for *Ming Pao*, which also thematically prioritises reporting on suicide, which is uniformly dramatic. This occurs despite *Ming Pao's* esteemed media reputation in Hong Kong for reliable, measured reporting, amidst an array of commercially successful competitors that are renowned for their unreserved, tabloid style of reporting (*BBC Monitoring* 2016). By contrast, the *People's Daily* rarely reports on suicide. It reports on suicide at a lower rate than it reports on crime. This comparative underreporting of suicide by the *People's Daily* is most likely due to the same reason it comparatively underreports on crime.

Reporting in all three newspapers thematically prioritises the celebrity experience of severe mental illness. The *Ming Pao* reports give as much attention to this experience as they give to that of everyday people. Moreover, the *Liberty Times* and the *People's Daily* reports give much greater attention to this experience than they give to that of everyday people. Indeed, the *People's Daily* never reports on lay people's everyday experience of severe mental illness. As a result, readers of *Liberty Times* and the *People's Daily* would more likely learn about what it is like to be a person with severe mental illness through the experiences of a "socially connected" celebrity, rather than an everyday fellow citizen (Olstead 2002, p. 640. See also Harper 2009). The commercial value of the celebrity voice can explain the relative prioritisation of the celebrity experience in the *Ming Pao* and *Liberty Times* reports. This, however, does not explain its relative prioritisation in their *People's Daily* counterparts. The detailed discourse analysis of these news reports in the upcoming chapters will shed more light on this.

Ming Pao and *Liberty Times* thematically prioritise reporting on crime where severe mental illness is implicated, while deprioritising that on politics, policy, and activism in severe mental illness. The *People's Daily* does the opposite, albeit not reporting on activism in any form. This likely reflects its status as the official messenger for the Communist Party and the mainland Chinese government. As such, politics takes priority over sensationalism and commercial value. Interestingly, medical reports comprise its foremost thematic category, in distinction to *Ming Pao* and *Liberty Times*. An explanation for this, too, requires more detailed discourse-level analysis in the upcoming chapters.

There are five outlier reports on severe mental illness across the three newspaper corpora. Two *Liberty Times* reports deal with missing persons (both women) who suffer from a severe mental illness. Another *Liberty Times* report points out the recent financial success of psychiatric pharmaceutical stocks in Taiwan. One *People's Daily* report examines education stress and severe mental illness, while another discusses the historical connection between European art and severe mental illness.

The reporting across the three Chinese-language newspapers numerically varies according to illness. Ninety-eight percent of reports nominally focus on one illness, with just 2% reporting on more than one illness. *Liberty Times* reports on depression around twice as much as *Ming Pao* and the *People's Daily* do. *Ming Pao* reports on schizophrenia and related psychoses around three times as much as *Liberty Times* and the *People's Daily* do. As such, *Ming Pao* proportionally overreports on schizophrenia and related psychoses, given the relative prevalence of such illness in comparison to depression (around 1:10). By contrast, *Liberty Times* reports on schizophrenia and depression proportionally in line with the relative prevalence of these illnesses in society. Around one half of the *Ming Pao* and *People's Daily* reports solely deal with generic severe mental illness, while less than one in six *Liberty Times* reports do. Georgaca and Bilić (2007) state that naming mental illnesses by using the generic expression rather than their specific diagnostic label "consolidate[s] [...] the difference between normality and abnormality" (p. 175). This adds to the contrast "between Us (the world) and Them (the mentally ill)" (Olstead 2002, p. 629).

Well over half of the *Ming Pao* and *Liberty Times* reports appear in the local – that is, Hong Kong regional or Taiwan regional – news section of the newspaper, in contrast to the *People's Daily* reports. The vast majority of reporting on severe mental illness in the *People's Daily* appears as ancillary specialist news. As such, it is less likely to be read by the lay reader. While the *Liberty Times* reports far outnumber their *Ming Pao* and *People's Daily* counterparts, they, on average, are much shorter in length. This, together with the *People's Daily* reports covering a year-long time period, as opposed to the six-month period for their *Ming Pao* and *Liberty Times* counterparts, results in the total character count for each of the three newspaper corpora closely aligning.

Chapter summary

This chapter outlines the social status of severe mental illness in the three culturally Chinese societies under study, namely, mainland China, Hong Kong, and Taiwan. The chapter sets out the criteria used to choose a leading Chinese-language newspaper from each geographical location, namely, audience reach, media reputation, and local ownership and production. It identifies and thematically categorises, as per Paterson (2007), the broad topics of reports on severe mental illness, which have been published in these newspapers in recent times. Although ostensibly similar in overall patterning, the thematic categories of each newspaper vary numerically in distinct ways. Some thematic differences may be readily attributable to a newspaper's broader commercial concerns, or the degree to which its reporting is controlled by the governing authorities. The chapter, nevertheless, points out that a more detailed discourse-level analysis can additionally explicate and explain any differences in reporting on severe mental illness across the three newspaper corpora in more informative and enlightening ways.

Chapters 3, 4, and 5 carry out such analyses. In so doing, the chapters clearly and transparently identify how and why the three leading Chinese-language newspapers selectively draw on, fortify, or contest the salient cultural, political, and institutional discourses in play in the three culturally Chinese societies under study. Framed by this chapter's thematic categorisation of the news reports, the discourse level analyses in Chapters 3, 4, and 5 explore, in greater detail, the extent to which, how, and why these reports

- equate severe mental illness to criminality and social wrongdoing.
- narrate people's life stories of severe mental illness.
- biomedicalise severe mental illness.
- co-opt it for political or activist gain.

In this way, the analyses in Chapters 3, 4, and 5 further evaluate the extent to which the construction of severe mental illness in the *People's Daily*, *Ming Pao* and *Liberty Times* news reports

- endorses or contests the dominant cultural, political, and biomedical narratives circulating in a geographical community.
- bears out or counters the intense stigma against severe mental illness in Chinese societies across the globe.
- empowers, includes, and humanises those with the illness.
- challenges and, so, potentially transforms a lay reader's "habits of mind" or "sets of fixed assumptions and expectations" in relation to severe mental illness (Gibson & Jacobson 2018, p. 187).

Note

1 The expression, United Front [统一战线], denotes the cooperative partnership between the ruling Communist Party and a number of legal minor parties and organisations that advocate for certain groups that make up greater Chinese society. Here, the relevant news article reports on the Taiwan Democratic Self-Government League [台湾民主自治同盟] (#10).

References

Angermeyer, M. C., & Schulze, B. (2001). Reinforcing stereotypes: How the focus on forensic cases in news reporting may influence public attitudes towards the mentally ill. *International Journal of Law and Psychiatry, 24*(4), 469–486.

Baum, E. (2018). *The invention of madness: State, society, and the insane in modern China*. Chicago: University of Chicago Press.

BBC Monitoring Asia Pacific. (2016, 12 September). Hong Kong media facing credibility crisis, survey shows. London, UK. https://search.proquest.com/docview/1818284777?accountid=14723

BBC News. (2013, 11 January). Q&A: China's newspaper industry. *BBC Online*. www.bbc.com/news/business-20970543.

Brady, A. (2002). Regimenting the public mind: The modernization of propaganda in the PRC. *International Journal, 57*(4), 563–578.

Brady, A. (2008). *Marketing dictatorship: Propaganda and thought work in contemporary China*. Lanham, MD: Rowman & Littlefield.

Brady, A. (2009). Mass persuasion as a means of legitimation and China's popular authoritarianism. *American Behavioral Scientist, 53*(3), 434–457.

Cao, Q. (2014). Introduction: Legitimisation, resistance and discursive struggles in contemporary China. In Q. Cao, H. Tian, & P. A. Chilton (Eds.), *Discourse, politics and media in contemporary China* (pp. 1–24). Amsterdam: John Benjamins.

Chan, K. Y., Zhao, F., Meng, S., Demaio, A. R., Reed, C., Theodoratou, E., Campbell, H., Wang, W., & Rudan, I. (2015). Prevalence of schizophrenia in China between 1990 and 2010. *Journal of Global Health, 5*(1), 1–8.

Chen, Y. M. (2011). The ideological construction of solidarity in translated newspaper commentaries: Context models and inter-subjective positioning. *Discourse and Society, 22*(6), 693–722.

Chen, Y., Yip, P. S. F., Tsai, C., & Fan, H. (2012). Media representation of gender patterns of suicide in Taiwan. *Crisis: The Journal of Crisis Intervention and Suicide Prevention, 33*(3), 144–150.

Chiu, M. L. (1981). Insanity in imperial China: A legal case study. In A. Kleinman & T. Lin (Eds.), *Normal and abnormal behaviour in Chinese culture* (pp. 75–94). Boston: D. Reidel.

Chiu, M. L. (1986). *Mind, body, and illness in a Chinese medical tradition* [Doctoral dissertation, Harvard University].

Chou, J. Y. (2006). *The psychiatric politics of risk and cost: Forensic theory and practice in the US and Taiwan* [Doctoral dissertation, University of Washington].

Choy, H. Y. F. (2016). Introduction: Disease and discourse. In H. Y. F. Choy (Ed.), *Discourses of disease: Writing illness, the mind and the body in modern China* (pp. 1–15). Leiden: Brill.

Corbin, J. M., & Strauss, A. L. (2008). *Basics of qualitative research: Techniques and procedures for developing grounded theory* (3rd ed.). Thousand Oaks, CA: SAGE.

Dikötter, F. (1998). *Imperfect conceptions: Medical knowledge, birth defects and eugenics in China*. London: Hurst & Co.

Every-Palmer, S., Brink, J., Chern, T. P., Choi, W. K., Hern-Yee, J. G., Green, B., Heffernan, E., Johnson, S. B., Kachaeva, M., Shiina, A., Walker, D., Wu, K., Wang, X., & Mellsop, G. (2014). Review of psychiatric services to mentally disordered offenders around the Pacific Rim. *Asia-Pacific Psychiatry, 6*(1), 1–17.

Fan, R., & Wang, M. (2015). Taking the role of the family seriously in treating Chinese psychiatric patients: A Confucian familist review of China's first mental health act. *The Journal of Medicine and Philosophy: A Forum for Bioethics and Philosophy of Medicine, 40*(4), 387–399.

Fu, T. S. T., Lee, C. S., Gunnell, D., Lee, W. C., & Cheng, A. T. A. (2013). Changing trends in the prevalence of common mental disorders in Taiwan: A 20-year repeated cross-sectional survey. *The Lancet, 381*(9862), 235–241.

Gallois, C., & Callan, V. J. (1997). *Communication and culture: A guide for practice.* Chichester: John Wiley & Sons.

Georgaca, E., & Bilić, B. (2007). Representations of "mental illness" in Serbian newspapers: A critical discourse analysis. *Qualitative Research in Psychology, 4*(1), 167–186.

Gibson, C., & Jacobson, T. (2018). Habits of mind in an uncertain information world. *Reference and User Services Quarterly, 57*(3), 183–192.

Guo, J. (2016). *Stigma: An ethnography of mental illness and HIV/AIDS in China.* Hackensack, NJ: World Century.

Han, D. Y., Lin, Y. Y., Liao, S. C., Lee, M. B., Thornicroft, G., & Wu, C. Y. (2015). Analysis of the barriers of mental distress disclosure in medical inpatients in Taiwan. *The International Journal of Social Psychiatry, 61*(5), 446–455.

Harper, S. (2009. *Madness, power and the media: Class, gender and race in popular representations of mental distress.* Basingstoke, UK: Palgrave Macmillan.

Heifetz, J. (2016, 28 June). Hong Kong's mental health crisis. *The Diplomat.* https://thediplomat.com/2016/06/hong-kongs-mental-health-crisis/

Ho, A. H. Y., Potash, J. S., Fong, T. C. T., Ho, V. F. L., Chen, E. Y. H., Lau, R. H. W., Au Yeung, F. S. W., & Ho, R. T. H. (2015). Psychometric properties of a Chinese version of the Stigma Scale: Examining the complex experience of stigma and its relationship with self-esteem and depression among people living with mental illness in Hong Kong. *Comprehensive Psychiatry, 56*(2015), 198–205.

Hsueh-Shih, C. (1995). Development of mental health systems and care in China: From the 1940s through the 1980s. In T. Lin, W. Tseng, & E. Yeh (Eds.), *Chinese society and mental health* (pp. 315–325). Hong Kong: Oxford University Press.

Hu, X., Rohrbaugh, R., Deng, Q., He, Q., Munger, K., & Liu, Z. (2017). Expanding the mental health workforce in China: Narrowing the mental health service gap. *Psychiatric Services, 68* (10), 987–989.

Hung, S. F. (2008). Hong Kong. Asia-Pacific community mental health development project report. www.wpanet.org/uploads/Examplary_Experiences/Asia-Pacific-Examplary-Experiences.pdf .

Jones, C. (1990). *Promoting prosperity: The Hong Kong way of social policy.* Hong Kong: Chinese University Press.

Kesic, D., Ducat, L. V., & Thomas, S. D. (2012). Using force: Australian newspaper depictions of contacts between the police and persons experiencing mental illness. *Australian Psychologist, 47* (4), 213–223.

Kleinman, A. (1986). *Social origins of distress and disease: Depression, neurasthenia, and pain in modern China.* London: Yale University Press.

Kleinman, A., Yan, Y., Jun, J., Lee, S., Zhang, E., Pan, T., Wu, F., & Guo, J. (2011). *Deep China: The moral life of the person: What anthropology and psychiatry tell us about China today.* Berkeley, CA: University of California Press.

Kuo, C. T. (2008). *Religion and democracy in Taiwan.* Albany, NY: SUNY Press.

Lee, H. W. (2015). From control to competition: A comparative study of the party press and popular press. In G. D. Rawnsley & M. T. Rawnsley (Eds.), *Routledge handbook of Chinese media* (pp. 117–130). New York: Routledge.

Li, G., Gutheil, T. G., & Hu, Z. (2016). Comparative study of forensic psychiatric system between China and America. *International Journal of Law and Psychiatry, 47*(2016), 164–170.

Lin, T. (1985). Mental disorders and psychiatry in Chinese culture: Characteristic features and major issues. In W. Tseng, & D. Y. H. Wu (Eds, *Chinese culture and mental health* (pp. 369–390). London: Academic Press.

Liu, J. (2008). *China.* Asia-Pacific community mental health development project report. www.wpanet.org/uploads/Examplary_Experiences/Asia-Pacific-Examplary-Experiences.pdf

Liu, S., & Page, A. (2016). Reforming mental health in China and India. *The Lancet, 388*(10042), 314–316.

Lo, L. K. (2011). Taiwan, Hong Kong, Macao. In P. C. Phan (Ed.), *Christianities in Asia* (pp. 173–183). Maldan, MA: Wiley-Blackwell.

Lu, C., Tung, C., & Ely, L. (2016). Reflection on the differences and similarities of mental health care in Virginia and Taiwan: Geography, history, culture, and nurse practitioners. *The Journal of Nursing, 63*(6), 107–113.

Mak, W. (1991). Mental health services in Hong Kong: History, modern development, and issues. *Journal of Sociology and Social Welfare, 18*(2), 127–139.

Mann, S. K. F., & Chong, B. B. W. (2016). How stigma from the public and significant others affects self-perception in people with mental illness in Hong Kong: A qualitative study. *Hong Kong Journal of Social Work, 50*(1/2), 3–25.

Mellor, D., Carne, L., Shen, Y. C., McCabe, M., & Wang, L. (2013). Stigma toward mental illness. *Journal of Cross-Cultural Psychology, 44*(3), 352–364.

Mendelson, D., & Lin, N. (2016). Mental health legislation (civil) in Australia and China: A comparative perspective. *Journal of Law and Medicine, 23*(4), 762–779.

Ng, V. W. (1990). *Madness in late imperial China: From illness to deviance.* London: University of Oklahoma Press.

Olstead, R. (2002). Contesting the text: Canadian media depictions of the conflation of mental illness and criminality. *Sociology of Health and Illness, 24*(5), 621–643.

Patel, V., Xiao, S., Chen, H., Hanna, F., Jotheeswaran, A. T., Luo, D., Parikh, R., Sharma, E., Usmani, S., Yu, Y., Druss, B. G., & Saxena, S. (2016). The magnitude of and health system responses to the mental health treatment gap in adults in India and China. *The Lancet, 388*(10063), 3074–3084.

Paterson, B. (2007). A discourse analysis of the construction of mental illness in two UK newspapers from 1985–2000. *Issues in Mental Health Nursing, 28*(10), 1087–1103.

Pearson, V. (1991). The development of modern psychiatric services in China 1891–1949. *History of Psychiatry, 2*(2), 133–147.

Pearson, V. (1992). Law, rights and psychiatry in the People's Republic of China. *International Journal of Law and Psychiatry, 15*, 409–423.

Pearson, V. (1996). The Chinese equation in mental health policy and practice. *International Journal of Law and Psychiatry, 19*(3/4), 437–458.

Peng, W., & Tang, L. (2010). Health content in Chinese newspapers. *Journal of Health Communication, 15*(7), 695–711.

Phillips, M., Chen, H., Diesfeld, K., Xie, B., Cheng, H., Mellsop, G., & Liu, X. (2013). China's new mental health law: Reframing involuntary treatment. *American Journal of Psychiatry, 170*(6), 588–591.

Ramsay, G. (2008). *Shaping minds: A discourse analysis of Chinese-language community mental health literature*. Amsterdam: John Benjamins.

Ramsay, G. (2013). *Mental illness, dementia and family in China*. London: Routledge.

Ramsay, G. (2016). *Chinese stories of drug addiction: Beyond the opium dens*. New York: Routledge.

Ran, M., Xiang, M., Simpson, P., & Chan, C. L. (2005). *Family-based mental health care in rural China*. Hong Kong: Hong Kong University Press.

Rosenberg, A. (2018, 18 June). *Hiding my mental illness from my Asian family almost killed me: The silent shame of having a mental illness in a Chinese family*. Vox. www.vox.com/first-person/2018/6/18/17464574/asian-chinese-community-mental-health-illness.

Sandby-Thomas, P. (2014). "Stability overwhelms everything": Analysing the legitimating effect of the stability discourse since 1989. In Q. Cao, H. Tian, & P. A. Chilton (Eds.), *Discourse, politics and media in contemporary China* (pp. 47–76). Amsterdam: John Benjamins.

Schiffrin, D. (1994). *Approaches to discourse*. Oxford: Blackwell.

Shepherd, C. (2017, 8 June). *China closes 60 celebrity gossip social media accounts*. Reuters. www.reuters.com/article/us-china-internet-censorship-idUSKBN18Z0J3.

Shi-xu. (2014). *Chinese discourse studies*. Hampshire, UK: Palgrave Macmillan.

Shi-xu. (2015). Towards a cultural methodology of human communication research: A Chinese example. In L. Tsung, & W. Wang (Eds.), *Contemporary Chinese discourse and social practice in China* (pp. 45–58). Amsterdam: John Benjamins.

Tong, J. (2014). Discourse of journalism and legitimacy in post-reform China. In Q. Cao, H. Tian, & P. A. Chilton (Eds.), *Discourse, politics and media in contemporary China* (pp. 123–144). Amsterdam: John Benjamins.

Topiwala, A., Wang, X., & Fazel, S. (2012). Chinese forensic psychiatry and its wider implications. *Journal of Forensic Psychiatry and Psychology, 23*(1), 1–6.

Traphagan. J. W. (2000). *Taming oblivion: Aging bodies and the fear of senility in Japan*. New York: State University of New York Press.

Tseng, W. (1973a). The development of psychiatric concepts in traditional Chinese medicine. *Archives of General Psychiatry, 29*(4), 569–575.

Tseng, W. (1973b). Concept of personality in Confucian thought. *Psychiatry, 36*(2), 191–202.

Tseng, W. (1986). Chinese psychiatry: Development and characteristics. In J. L. Cox (Ed.), *Transcultural psychiatry* (pp. 274–290). London: Crown Helm.

van Dijk, T. A. (1988a). *News analysis: Case studies of international and national news in the press*. Hillsdale, NJ: Lawrence Erlbaum.

Wahl, O., Wood, A., & Richards, R. (2002). Newspaper coverage of mental illness: Is it changing? *Psychiatric Rehabilitation Skills, 6*(1), 9–31.

Wang, W., & Liu, Y. (2016). Discussing mental illness in Chinese social media: The impact of influential sources on stigmatization and support among their followers. *Health Communication, 31*(3), 355–363.

World Health Organization. (2011). *Mental health atlas 2011: China, Hong Kong Special Administrative Region*. Geneva: Department of Mental Health and Substance Abuse, World Health Organization.

Wu, E. C. H. (2008). *Taiwan*. Asia-Pacific community mental health development project report. www.wpanet.org/uploads/Examplary_Experiences/Asia-Pacific-Examplary-Experiences.pdf

Wu, H. Y. J., & Cheng, A. T. A. (2017). A history of mental healthcare in Taiwan. In H. Minas, & M. Lewis (Eds.), *Mental health in Asia and the Pacific: Historical and cultural perspectives* (pp. 107–121). Boston, MA: Springer.

Xia, Z., & Zhang, M. (1981). History and present status of modern psychiatry in China. *Chinese Medical Journal, 94*(5), 277–282.

Xu, X., Li, X. M., Xu, D., & Wang, W. (2017). Psychiatric and mental health nursing in China: Past, present and future. *Archives of Psychiatric Nursing, 31*(5), 470–476.

Xue, L., Shi, Y. W., Knoll, J., & Zhao, H. (2015). Chinese forensic psychiatry: History, development and challenges. *Journal of Forensic Science and Medicine, 1*(1), 61–67.

Yan, H. (1985). Some psychological problems manifested by neurotic patients: Shanghai examples. In W. Tseng & D. Y. H. Wu (Eds.), *Chinese culture and mental health* (pp. 325–338). London: Academic Press.

Yang, Y., & Parrott, S. (2018). Schizophrenia in Chinese and U.S. online news media: Exploring cultural influence on the mediated portrayal of schizophrenia. *Health Communication, 33*(5), 553–561.

Yip, K. S. (1998). A historical review of mental health services in Hong Kong (1841 to 1995). *International Journal of Social Psychiatry, 44*(1), 46–55.

Zhang, Y., Jin, Y., & Tang, Y. (2015). Framing depression: Cultural and organizational influences on coverage of a public health threat and attribution of responsibilities in Chinese news media, 2000–2012. *Journalism and Mass Communication Quarterly, 92*(1), 99–120.

Zhuang, X. Y., Wong, D. F. K., Cheng, C. W., & Pan, S. M. (2017). Mental health literacy, stigma and perception of causation of mental illness among Chinese people in Taiwan. *International Journal of Social Psychiatry, 63*(6), 498–507.

3   Severe mental illness as crime and social wrongdoing

The previous chapter has identified that news reports on crime and suicide thematically dominate the reporting on severe mental illness in *Ming Pao* and *Liberty Times*. The *People's Daily*, by contrast, thematically deprioritises reports of this type. This chapter examines how these leading Chinese-language newspapers discursively construct severe mental illness as crime and social wrongdoing such as ignominious suicide. The chapter discusses available contemporary data on forensic psychiatric crime and suicide across greater China. This provides a social context for the detailed discourse-level analysis that follows on from these discussions. The analysis follows the approach set out in the Chapter 1 section on the analysis of Chinese-language print media reports on severe mental illness. This approach provides nuanced and in-depth comparative insights into how the Chinese-language newspapers under study report on severe mental illness and why they do so in the ways they do (Kesic, Ducat, & Thomas 2012; Knifton & Quinn 2008; Olstead 2002; van Dijk 1988a).

Forensic psychiatric crime in present-day greater China

It is unavoidable that data on the level of crime where severe mental illness is implicated in present-day mainland China, Hong Kong, and Taiwan will be incomplete and indeterminate. This is because such data is only collected where a crime of this type has come to the attention of judicial agencies or their affiliates. Crime such as domestic violence perpetrated by or against those with a severe mental illness may often go unreported. This is especially so in Chinese societies, where public revelation of such crime, in addition to public disclosure of severe mental illness in a family, can bring about great loss of face. Despite the obvious limitations of published data, tentative claims can still be made about the level of forensic psychiatric crime in present-day greater China, by examining a range of contemporary data from diverse sources.

Li, Gutheil, and Hu (2016) record that there were 57,513 forensic psychiatric assessments carried out in mainland Chinese mental health facilities in 2014. Here, forensic means relating to the law or legal processes. In mainland

China, forensic psychiatric assessments can be initiated by the courts or public security forces (Li, Gutheil, & Hu 2016). While the number of these assessments is high, it, of course, stems from a large population base on the mainland. Li, Gutheil, and Hu (2016, p. 168) add that mainland China had 25 "*Ankang* (security and recovery)" [安康] hospitals in 2005, totalling more than 7,000 forensic psychiatric beds. Topiwala, Wang, and Fazel (2012) and Every-Palmer, Brink, Chern et al. (2014) record similar numbers of *Ankang* hospitals and forensic psychiatric beds in mainland China in 2012. This puts the per capita number of forensic psychiatric beds in mainland China at one-fifth of that in the U.K. (Topiwala, Wang, & Fazel 2012).

Ankang hospitals intern perpetrators of crime who have a severe mental illness and cannot be held criminally responsible for their misdeeds (Li, Gutheil, & Hu 2016). Topiwala, Wang, and Fazel (2012) and Every-Palmer, Brink, Chern et al. (2014), nevertheless, state that *Ankang* hospitals only intern a portion of these perpetrators. A large number of them remain housed in the local mental health facilities that the police initially send them to, or are returned to their families for care and supervision (Every-Palmer, Brink, Chern et al. 2014; Li, Gutheil, & Hu 2016; Xue, Shi, Knoll et al. 2015). As is the case for all people with a severe mental illness in mainland China, the family is legally responsible for their care and supervision in the local community (Every-Palmer, Brink, Chern et al. 2014; Li, Gutheil, & Hu 2016; Phillips, Chen, Diesfeld et al. 2013; Topiwala, Wang, & Fazel 2012; Xue, Shi, Knoll et al. 2015). This includes those who commit a crime, but are benevolently (or in institutional self-interest) released back to their families. Somewhat alarmingly, yet unsurprising given the intense stigma against severe mental illness in Chinese culture (Guo 2016; Kleinman, Yan, Jun et al. 2011; Ramsay 2013; Wang & Liu 2016; Xu, Li, Xu et al. 2017), most mentally ill perpetrators of crime who are returned to the care and supervision of their families in mainland China do not receive any follow-up psychiatric care (Every-Palmer, Brink, Chern et al. 2014). Xue, Shi, Knoll et al. (2015) record an official total of 40,822 mentally ill perpetrators of crime in mainland China in 2010. This aligns with Li, Gutheil, and Hu's (2016) figure for forensic psychiatric assessments in 2016. However, Xue, Shi, Knoll et al.'s (2015) official figure likely only accounts for *Ankang* internments. Adding the large number of mentally ill perpetrators of crime who are housed in local mental health facilities or returned to their families for care and supervision to Xue, Shi, Knoll et al.'s (2015) figure would likely generate a total of around 100,000 people or more, a per capita rate of approximately one in ten thousand on the mainland.

While mainland China has around 25 dedicated forensic psychiatric facilities, Hong Kong has just one, Siu Lam Psychiatric Centre [小欖精神病治療中心] (Chan & Chow 2014; Every-Palmer, Brink, Chern et al. 2014). Siu Lam Psychiatric Centre is located in a remote part of the New Territories of the Hong Kong Special Administrative Region. It has a 261-bed capacity for male and female prisoners who suffer from a severe mental illness (Hong Kong Correctional Services 2018). Chan and Chow (2014) report that

Siu Lam Psychiatric Centre carried out 343 court-ordered forensic psychiatric assessments over a six-month period in 2012, of which 76.4% were for men with a severe mental illness and 23.6% were for women with such illness. An annual figure of several hundred cases of forensic psychiatric crime in Hong Kong would produce a per capita figure that broadly aligns with that for mainland China, namely around one in ten thousand.

Taiwan has no dedicated forensic psychiatric hospitals like *Ankang* and Siu Lam Psychiatric Centre. It does, however, have two dedicated prisons that are expressly set up for offenders with a severe mental illness (Every-Palmer, Brink, Chern et al. 2014). These, of course, are penal units, not hospitals. Every-Palmer, Brink, Chern et al. (2014) state that most offenders who have a severe mental illness in Taiwan are treated in mental health units of local hospitals and then sent on to regular prisons. Wu, Chou, Yeh et al. (2017) state that district-level courts across Taiwan referred 3,467 people for forensic psychiatric examination between 2002 and 2010, approximately 450 referrals per year on average. Every-Palmer, Brink, Chern et al. (2014, p. 11), however, caution that people with a severe mental illness who are standing trial in Taiwan are only referred for "forensic psychiatric examination [...] in difficult cases following the court approval" (see also Wu, Chou, Yeh et al. 2017; Yang, Yu, & Pan 2017). Judges can choose not to refer such cases (Wu, Chou, Yeh et al. 2017; Yang, Yu, & Pan 2017). However, if they do refer them, they "have the final authority to accept or not accept the forensic psychiatrists' professional opinions" (Wu, Chou, Yeh et al. 2017, p. 321).

The Judicial Yuan of the Republic of China (2018) records that, between 2015 and 2017, thousands of cases where severe mental illness was implicated were heard each year across all levels of courts in Taiwan. On average, around 200 such cases were heard each year by the Supreme Court in Taiwan, which is the highest court in the land; while around 830 such cases were heard each year by the array of High Courts in Taiwan (Judicial Yuan of the Republic of China 2018). The High Courts in Taiwan are subordinate to the Supreme Court. These figures point to an annual rate of forensic psychiatric crime in Taiwan that aligns with, or exceeds, that for mainland China and Hong Kong.

Thus, based on an array of contemporary data, it appears that the level of crime where severe mental illness is implicated does not vary markedly across greater China. The level of such crime in Taiwan, in fact, may be somewhat higher than its counterparts across the straits. As a result, the proportionally lower reporting on crime where severe mental illness is implicated in *Liberty Times*, as compared to *Ming Pao*, appears to be discursively significant. Likewise, the proportionally lower reporting on such crime in the *People's Daily*, when compared to *Ming Pao* and *Liberty Times*, also appears to be significant. The *People's Daily* may deliberately underreport such crime relative to *Ming Pao* and *Liberty Times* (Zhang 2019). This is because, to do otherwise may undermine the oft-made claim by the party and the state that they are successfully maintaining social harmony and social stability [维和维稳] on the mainland. On the other hand, *Liberty Times*, unlike *Ming*

Pao, may knowingly curtail reporting on crime where severe mental illness is implicated. The newspaper may magnanimously avoid exploiting the sensational and, so, commercial value of reporting on it, in consideration of people with a severe mental illness. The following detailed discourse-level analysis of the crime reports in the *People's Daily*, *Ming Pao*, and *Liberty Times* will add weight to or challenge such claims.

Crime reports

Approximately two-thirds of the *People's Daily* and *Ming Pao* crime reports deal with violent crime where people with a severe mental illness are the perpetrators. Just over one-half of the *Liberty Times* crime reports do so. Across all three newspapers, the vast majority of these mentally ill perpetrators are men. An additional 20% of the *Ming Pao* crime reports and an additional 12% of the *Liberty Times* crime reports deal with non-violent crime where people with a severe mental illness are the perpetrators. Most of these mentally ill perpetrators are women in the *Ming Pao* reports, while all of them are men in the *Liberty Times* counterparts. Almost one-third of the *Liberty Times* crime reports, yet only one in twelve of their *Ming Pao* counterparts, deal with violent crime where people with a severe mental illness are the victims. There is gender parity for these victims in the *Ming Pao* reports. By contrast, all but one of these victims are women in the *Liberty Times* reports. The remaining crime reports in the three newspapers are very few in number, and deal with non-violent crime where people with a severe mental illness are the victims (three men and one woman); or non-violent crime committed by mentally well people who have a family member with a severe mental illness (one man and one woman).

Most of the crime reports are published in the local news sections of the newspapers, which are more likely to be read by readers (see Appendices 1–3). The *Ming Pao* reports are published quite evenly across each month for the six-month period of analysis, while their *Liberty Times* counterparts cluster in January, March, and June (see Appendices 2 and 3). No single news event contributes to this cluster, including the brutal random killing of a young girl in Taipei in late March. There are only three *People's Daily* crime reports published over an extended twelve-month period of analysis (see Appendix 1). While approximately two-thirds of the *Ming Pao* and *People's Daily* crime reports deal with generic severe mental illness, more than two-thirds of the *Liberty Times* crime reports deal with depression (see Appendices 1–3).

Crime committed by people with a severe mental illness, therefore, attracts a lot of coverage in both *Ming Pao* and *Liberty Times*, with very little coverage in the *People's Daily*. There is greater coverage in *Ming Pao* than in *Liberty Times*. The coverage in *Liberty Times* further differs from that in *Ming Pao* in giving greater attention to people with a severe mental illness who are victims of crime. Nearly all of the reported victims are women. This reporting in the *Liberty Times* is more in line with the fact that people with a severe mental illness are more likely to be victims of crime than perpetrators of crime (Cashman & Thomas 2017; Hsu, Sheu, Liu et al. 2009; Rukavina, Nawka, Brborović et al. 2012; Varshney, Mahapatra, Krishnan et al. 2016). Reporting in the *Liberty Times* also differs from that in *Ming Pao* by routinely specifying the name of the severe mental illness, here, depression. *Ming Pao* mostly uses the generic label severe mental illness. Georgaca and Bilić (2007, p. 175) state that use of the generic label bolsters, in a disempowering way, the rudimentary distinction between "normal" mentally well citizens and "abnormal" mentally ill ones.

The headline of a news report constitutes the highest level of its superstructural hierarchy (van Dijk 1988a, 1988b). As such, the semantic and finer linguistic features of a headline hold a high degree of discursive prominence and import. The *Ming Pao* and *People's Daily* crime reports commonly call attention to the link between severe mental illness and crime by making mention of the illness in their headlines. This is particularly so in violent crime. The *Ming Pao* headlines not only foreground the link between severe mental illness and violent crime, they further name perpetrators, in an essentialising way, using an illness label (see selected Examples 1–3).

1. Attacks Diners With Fake Gun – <u>Schizophrenic Woman</u> Sentenced With Hospitalisation Order[1] [假槍襲食客 精神分裂婦判醫院令] (#45)[2]
2. <u>Mentally Ill Man</u> Bashes Victim's Head During Robbery – Jailed For 5 Years 9 Months [精神病漢扑頭搶劫 囚5年9月] (#70)
3. <u>Psychiatric Hospital Patient</u> Chases, Knifes Woman Passer-By – After Assault Wanders Around – Arrested On Return To Rehab Centre [精神病院友追斬女途人 行兇後遊蕩 返復康中心被拘] (#77)

Naming people in this way defines them by way of their illness. This is because linguistically there is no clear separation between their personhood and their illness. The Chinese language can express such a separation, just as English can through the use of a relative clause. The *Ming Pao* headlines further position the mentally ill perpetrators of crime as agents of verbs that denote negative, aggressive action. They "attack" [襲], "gouge out" [挖掉], "rob" [劫], "slap"[摑], "bash" [扑], "stab" [刑], "knife" [斬], "chase" [追], or "conspire to murder" [串謀謀殺]. These actions are given prominence through their appearance in the opening clause of the headline. The headlines also identify the mentally well victims of these actions as someone known to the mentally ill perpetrator, usually an immediate family member; or, just as commonly, as someone unknown to the perpetrator, such as "diners" or "passers-by." Identifying the mentally well victim as someone who is unknown to the perpetrator points to the random nature of many of these violent offences. The headlines also commonly make clear that the mentally ill perpetrator is now detained in a hospital or prison. That is, they have been brought under control. Who effects this control is obscured by the use of passive voice, maintaining attention on the mentally ill perpetrator. Thus, within the short wording of a headline, the *Ming Pao* crime reports construct people with a severe mental illness as threatening beings consumed by an illness that makes them behave aggressively, even to strangers, such that they need to be removed safely away from everyday society.

The *People's Daily* headlines, although very few in number, also link severe mental illness to violent crime. They, however, do so in separate independent or adverbial clauses. This means that the mentally ill perpetrators are not named, in an essentialising way, through their illness. In Example 4 below, the headline, instead, names the perpetrator in a legalistic way, as a "suspect." This headline also maintains attention on the perpetrator, using nominalisation and passive voice to obscure who suspects him of murder, who arrested him, and who clinically assessed him as having depression. It similarly obscures his victim through its use of the generic legalistic expression, "case."

4. "Sichuan Normal University Bloody Murder <u>Case</u>" <u>Suspect</u> Teng <u>Arrested</u> – Previously <u>Identified</u> As Having Depression ["川师大血案"嫌疑人滕某被批捕 此前被鉴定为抑郁症] (#4)

The headlines of the *Liberty Times* crime reports, however, differ. They rarely name perpetrators of a violent crime by way of their illness or make mention of their illness at all (see selected Examples 5 and 6).

5. <u>25-Year-Old Woman</u> Robs Jewellery Store – Wounds 62-Year-Old Woman Right After Getting Bail [25歲女搶銀樓才交保 又殺傷62歲婦] (#117)
6. "If Child Murder Case Gets Light Sentence, <u>I</u> Will Do The Same!" – <u>Man</u> Arrested For Drunken Ravings [「殺童案輕判就模仿」男醉後狂言被逮] (#134)

As a result, the aggressive actions of the perpetrators, here, "robs," "wounds," and "do the same" (i.e., murder a child), are not proximately linked to severe mental illness. The agents of these verbs are denoted by way of everyday collective nouns and personal pronouns, namely "woman," "man," and "I." The headlines maintain focus on the perpetrators, even though not making any mention of their illness. Example 5 does not state who gave the perpetrator bail; and Example 6 does not state who arrested the perpetrator, or who would sentence the child murderer whom the perpetrator wishes to emulate. Furthermore, Example 6 impersonally and legalistically denotes this murderer as a "case."

In the rare instances where the *Liberty Times* headlines link severe mental illness to violent crime, they do so in ways similar to their *Ming Pao* and *People's Daily* counterparts (see Examples 7 and 8).

7. Younger Brother Slashes Older Brother With Watermelon Knife – <u>Claims To Have Severe Mental Illness</u> [弟拿西瓜刀砍傷兄 供稱精神病] (#100)

8. "Go Kill Someone!" – <u>Schizophrenic</u> Man Allegedly Hears Voices, Stabs Aunt To Death, Charged [「快去殺人」思覺失調男疑幻聽刺死姑姑被訴] (#150)

Example 7 links severe mental illness to violent crime by way of a separate independent clause. Example 8 names the mentally ill perpetrator, in an essentialising way, through his illness. It also maintains focus on him, by not naming who charges him or who alleges that he hears voices. Notably, the opening clause of the headline is an imperative statement that points to the potential unpredictability of his violence, which targets a seemingly arbitrary "someone," even though later on the headline reveals that his own family member was the victim.

Where violent crime involves sexual assault, the headlines of the *Ming Pao* and *Liberty Times* reports make no mention of severe mental illness. The circumstances of these sexual assaults, however, differ across these newspapers in that people with a severe mental illness tend to be the perpetrators of sexual assault in the *Ming Pao* reports, while they tend to be the victims in their *Liberty Times* counterparts. The headlines of these *Ming Pao* reports describe the perpetrators of a sexual assault not by their illness but by features that appear to reflect stereotypical, at times discriminatory, attitudes towards and beliefs about sexual assault: ethnic minority men hoodwink and molest dominant culture youth; male school workers rape school girls; troubled old men sexually molest young girls (see Examples 9–11).

9. Seizes Opportunity To Kiss Face, Has Oral Sex – <u>Pakistani Man</u> Pretends To Ask Directions, <u>Molests 2 Youth</u> [乘機吻臉口交巴漢扮問路狎兩青年] (#46)
10. <u>Naked Male Worker</u> Tries To <u>Rape Schoolgirl At School</u> [裸男工校內圖姦女生] (#62)
11. Claims Possessed, <u>Molests Little Girl</u> – <u>Old Man In 60s</u> Convicted With Hospitalisation Order [稱撞邪狎女童 六旬翁判醫院令] (#78)

Familiar sexual assault scripts, therefore, appear to supplant that of the violent mentally ill criminal in these headlines. At this highest level of the news text superstructural hierarchy, the sexual assault scripts may be more coherent to readers. Not only are the scripts familiar, but they invite the use of salacious and mystifying language that can attract the readers' attention (Angermeyer & Schulze 2001; Richardson 2007). The perpetrators "kiss," "have oral sex," "molest," "are naked," "rape," and "are possessed." The headlines give precedence to these lurid actions and states of being, placing them at clause-initial positions, or in the opening sentence of a two-sentence headline.

The headlines of the *Liberty Times* reports on sexual assault, by contrast, bear out their focus on people with a severe mental illness as victims, rather than perpetrators, of crime. In so doing, they gender the experience of victimhood in disempowering ways for the largely women victims (see selected Examples 12–14).

12. Drugs, Sexually Assaults <u>Young Girl</u> – She Jumps Off Building – Sentenced To 10 Years Jail, Fined 1 Million [餵毒性侵害少女跳樓判10年賠100萬] (#101)
13. Causes <u>Girlfriend</u> To Suicide – Dentist Gets Off Sexual Assault – 1 Year Jail For Grievous Bodily Harm [害女友輕生 牙醫性侵脫罪傷害囚1年] (#182)
14. Dislikes S&M Sex Worker – Client To Text <u>Her Children</u>, Forces <u>Her</u> To Submit [搞SM被嫌 嫖客電告她兒女逼就範] (#193)

Like many of the *Liberty Times* reports on other types of crime, these headlines make no mention of severe mental illness. Example 12 omits any mention of the (male) perpetrator. Discursive attention remains on the young girl. As victim, she is passively subject to lurid acts, namely "drugging" and "sexual assault," which are committed upon her by an unnamed assailant. These acts are foregrounded in the opening clause. She subsequently is given agency, but through a destructive, ignominious act of suicide. Example 13, likewise, omits the (male) perpetrator in the opening clause, placing focus on the girlfriend. Unlike the young girl in Example 13, the girlfriend lacks agency even in the destructive act of ignominious suicide. Her (at this stage) unnamed assailant "causes" her to suicide. The assailant is subsequently named by way of what is widely thought to be an upstanding profession. Thereafter, the victim's personhood is erased, being subsumed by the nominalised "sexual assault" and "grievous bodily harm." Nominalisation concomitantly removes the perpetrator's agency in the sexual assault, who, instead, is awarded somewhat more positive agency in "getting off." Example 14 further feminises sexual assault by drawing attention to the victim's motherhood, which, in Chinese culture, would plainly sit at odds with her prefaced profession of "S&M sex worker" (Croll 1995; Guo 2010). Once again, the (male) perpetrator of the crime is unnamed in the opening clause, yet gains agency through the largely unproblematic initial actions of "dislike" and "text." When first named, the perpetrator also is innocuously named as a "client," in contrast to the victim's salacious title of "S&M sex worker."

The headline of a *Liberty Times* report where a woman with a severe mental illness is the victim of domestic violence similarly genders the experience of victimhood in disempowering ways. The opening sentence of the headline calls attention to the woman's failed agency (see Example 15 below). This sentence is sequentially linked, or, more insidiously, causally linked, to the perpetrator's violence.

15. Wife <u>Fails</u> To Fix PC – Horror Husband First Beats Then Burns Her [妻修不好電腦 恐怖丈夫先揍後燒] (#184)

Once again, the headline of this *Liberty Times* crime report makes no mention of severe mental illness.

The headline of the sole *People's Daily* report on sexual assault deals with a male perpetrator with a severe mental illness. It innocuously names him as a "student" (see Example 16 below). It foregrounds that he is residing overseas, which distances his actions away from the domestic arena. By implication, this is not something that would happen in mainland China. The headline explicitly links his crime to severe mental illness, through a deferred adverbial clause of reason. This greater blaming of the illness, and doing so after naming the perpetrator in an innocuous way and locating him overseas, somewhat ameliorates his culpability for his crime, when compared to the discursive practices in the headline of the *People's Daily* murder report (see earlier Example 4). The latter headline opens with the crime; sensationally describes it as "bloody"; names the (male) perpetrator in a legalistic way; and maintains attention on him alone. The headline of the sexual assault report, however, names the victims as well as the perpetrator, and by way of identical designations, namely, "student." This directs attention to others, namely, the victims, and nominally personalises the perpetrator in the same way as them. Moreover, the personalised victims are further reduced to sexualised body parts, namely, their "thighs." This genders the experience of victimhood in disempowering ways, as the headlines of the *Liberty Times* crime reports often do.

16. Chinese <u>Student Studying Abroad In USA</u> Gropes <u>Female Students' Thighs</u> At Campus <u>Due To Severe Mental Illness</u> [中国留美学生因患精神病在校园乱摸女生大腿] (#21)

Across all three newspapers, reporting on non-violent crime is much less common than that on violent crime. *Ming Pao* reports the most on such crime. Interestingly, its reports make mention of severe mental illness as a mere segue to, or pretext for, discussion of wider concerns in contemporary society. Most of the headlines of these reports on non-violent crime do not make any mention of severe mental illness. Those that do illustrate how the illness can be used to draw attention to other wider social concerns. Example 17 below alludes to institutional malfeasance in Hong Kong, both within aged care facilities and the police. The victim is named, in an essentialising way, through her severe mental illness. She lacks agency, in that she is passively "coaxed"; and her money, rather than herself, is defrauded. This contrasts with the retirement home's active "embezzling," and the police who firmly "refuse" to take further action.

17. Retirement Home Involved In <u>Embezzling Mentally Ill Woman's 230,000 HKD</u> – <u>Coaxed</u> Into Signing Investment Contract – Police <u>Refuse</u> Further Investigation [安老院涉吞精神病婦23萬　勸誘簽署投資合約警拒深入調查] (#44)

Example 18 below, also from *Ming Pao*, alludes to institutional safeguard measures failing to prevent a man with a severe mental illness from fraudulently donating his sperm, which was subsequently used to produce a large number of children. The headline names the man, in essentialising ways, through his severe mental illness and his legal status as a "criminal." This conflates the illness and criminality. The headline also contrasts the deceitfulness of the man with a severe mental illness, who "pretends," with the apparent uprightness of a "scholar." In addition, it metonymically reduces the man with a severe mental illness, and his agency in "bearing" children, to the elemental cellular component of "sperm." This, together with the use of the expression "descendants," call to mind the biogenetic component to stigma against severe mental illness in Chinese culture, whereby the illness is deemed to pollute family lines (Dikötter 1998).

18. Mentally Ill Criminal Pretends To Be Scholar – Donated Sperm Bears 36 Descendants [精神病犯冒才子 捐精誕36後代] (#53)

In sum, the *Ming Pao* and *People's Daily* headlines discursively fortify the link between severe mental illness and crime, while the *Liberty Times* headlines do not. The discursive reach of this phenomenon is much greater in the case of *Ming Pao*, given its comparatively high number of crime reports. At this highest level of the news text superstructural hierarchy, the *Ming Pao* headlines not only frequently make mention of severe mental illness, but use it to name perpetrators and victims of crime, in essentialising ways. As such, people are reduced to their illness. These headlines also prominently locate verbs denoting the negative, aggressive actions of mentally ill perpetrators at clause-initial positions or in opening clauses. This is the case for the reports on violent crime in all three newspapers, regardless of whether they reveal the mental health status of the perpetrators. The sensational and, so, commercial value of doing so is clearly in play. Such language attracts a reader's attention. The *Ming Pao* headlines further call attention to the randomness of violent crime where severe mental illness is implicated in Hong Kong. Doing so would heighten the threat that people with such illness pose to the local community. Thus, the *Ming Pao* headlines appear to take full advantage of the sensational and, so, commercial value of crime where severe mental illness is implicated. They do so even when a crime is non-violent in nature, using it as a segue or pretext for discussion and critique of wider social concerns.

The headlines of all three newspapers maintain focus on the perpetrators of crime, regardless of their mental health status. Victims with a severe mental illness, on the other hand, are routinely cast as passive beings and prone to ignominious acts; or they are discursively erased. Nearly all the victims are women. The *Liberty Times* headlines deal with crime *against* people with a severe mental illness much more often than its counterparts do. This is more in line with the actual experience of crime in severe mental illness. While experientially more authentic, these headlines make clear that the victims, nearly all of whom are women, are known to the perpetrators of the crimes against them. This could perversely reduce the perceived public threat posed by such crime, given prejudicial gender discourses that espouse that women attract or precipitate attacks against them, especially when the perpetrators are known to them (Burnett, Mattern, Herakova et al. 2009; Cowan 2000; Suarez & Gadalla 2010).

The headline represents the highest level of the news text superstructural hierarchy. It gives discursive expression to a news report's overarching semantic and finer linguistic features. More detailed identification and understanding of the report's discursive practices require analysis of the sentences that make up its opening paragraph. This may be the lead paragraph or the reporting of the main event of a news story, in the absence of a lead paragraph. Nearly all of the news reports under study lack a discrete lead paragraph.

The schematic structure of the *Ming Pao* crime reports where severe mental illness is implicated is unique across the three newspapers. This is because most of them are rudimentary summaries of published court case documents. They are marked so with a "Case Number" in brackets, at the very end of the report, for example: "(Case Number: STCC1535/16)" [【案件編號：STCC1535/16】] (#46). As a result, the schematic structure of the *Ming Pao* crime reports is uniform and simple. The headlines are followed by details about what took place when a crime was committed, as well as the ensuing court case after the perpetrator is arrested by the authorities. The former content constitutes the main event of the news story, that is, the actual crime; while the latter content constitutes its consequences, that is, the sentencing of the perpetrator (van Dijk 1988a, 1988b). This narrow schematic structure discursively aligns with the most rudimentary of crime narratives. Perpetrators commit crime, are arrested, tried, sentenced, and imprisoned. As a result, the *Ming Pao* crime reports where severe mental illness is implicated would be readily identifiable as a crime report to a reader. Moreover, what is prioritised in the headlines of these reports is discursively coherent with their ensuing schematic structure. Where the schematic structure of the *Ming Pao* crime reports does not fully emulate that of an orthodox crime narrative, it still strongly bears out such a narrative. The consequences of a crime in one report are not legal proceedings but the public exposing of the perpetrator's Instagram account by irate internet users. The consequence in another report is intervention by the government medical disputes agency, since the perpetrator was a psychiatric hospital inpatient. Those in another report are the immediate hospitalisation of the pair of perpetrators on their arrest. All in all, there is no greater nuancing of, or greater divergence from, an orthodox crime narrative schema.

The schematic structure of the *Liberty Times* crime reports, by contrast, is more sophisticated than their *Ming Pao* counterparts. They are not rudimentary summaries of published court case documents. They also place greater discursive distance between people and their severe mental illness than their

Ming Pao counterparts do. The latter routinely name people, at this upper level of the news text superstructural hierarchy,

- through their illness, as the headlines do.
- using legalistic labels: "gunman" [槍手], "crime suspect" [疑犯/ 疑兇], "offender" [肇事者].
- by combining illness and legalistic labels: "mental illness[3] sufferer with a record of assault" [有傷人前科的精神病患者].
- through their low social status: "unemployed man" [無業漢], "unemployed woman" [無業婦].
- through their illness and low social status: "woman with schizophrenia and on welfare" [患有精神分裂領綜援婦人]; "father of 8 with illicit-drug-induced severe mental illness" [育有8名子女、曾因濫藥致精神病的父親].

By contrast, the opening paragraphs of the *Liberty Times* reports grammatically delink people from their severe mental illness, by using the Chinese qualifier particle *de* [的]. This functions like a "who" relative clause in English (see selected Examples 19 and 20 below). Despite these reports' greater distinction between individuals and their illness, they are awash with legalistic lexis and grammar, like their *Ming Pao* counterparts. They routinely state the family name of people with a severe mental illness immediately before the Chinese nominal classifier "to be named" [姓] (see selected Examples 19 and 20 below). In more colloquial language, the family name would appear immediately after this nominal classifier.

19. <u>a woman by the name of</u> Wang, <u>who</u> has severe depression [有重度憂鬱症的王姓婦人] (#107)
20. <u>a man by the name of</u> Chang, <u>who</u> suffers from schizophrenia [一名罹患思覺失調症的張姓男子] (#187)

They similarly state the family name of those with the illness immediately before the Chinese indefinite classifier "a certain" [某]; or state their family name immediately before the Chinese nominal classifier "to be a criminal suspect" [嫌]) (see selected Examples 21 and 22).

21. His family were all shocked that he had expressed remarks about doing a copycat murder of a child. They hastily explained to police that <u>a certain Mr Yun</u> suffers from severe mental illness, and makes erratic phone calls after getting drunk. [家人對於他發表仿效殺童言論都大吃一驚，趕緊向警方解釋雲某罹患精神病，酒醉後亂打電話。] (#134)
22. <u>Suspect Ling</u> denied that he is a drug dealer, claiming that he suffers from depression and needs to use illicit drugs to ease his mood and relieve stress. [凌嫌否認是毒梟辯稱他患有憂鬱症，需施用毒品來紓解情緒及解除壓力。] (#154)

Not only do Examples 21 and 22 rhetorically attribute the crimes committed by the legalistically named perpetrators to their severe mental illness, they also proximally link the illness to other social wrongdoing, such as illicit drug peddling and use, alcohol abuse, and "erratic" public behaviour. These examples further construct the mentally ill perpetrators in a legalistic way, by describing what they say as an "expressed remark," "denial," and "claim." Mentally well family members, by contrast, informatively "explain," as everyday people do (see Example 21). In addition, Example 21 diminishes the agency of the mentally ill perpetrator by describing his intended crime as a "copycat" action rather than one of his own conception. Example 22 also modally casts illicit drug use, in detrimental and disempowering ways, as something that those with depression "need to" do. As a result, depression is correlated to illicit drug use, a highly transgressive act that people with depression are driven to rather than choose to do.

Examples 23 and 24 below are typical opening paragraphs of *Ming Pao* and *Liberty Times* crime reports, respectively.

23. Following on from a mental illness sufferer wielding a knife on the street and "indiscriminately" chasing and knifing women passers-by in Tai Kok Tsui on the 26th of last month, a "copycat" bloody crime has again taken place in Yuen Long. Yesterday, a mental illness sufferer with a record of assault attacked two women passers-by on the street with a box cutter, then discarded the knife and walked away as if nothing had happened. Fortunately, an enthusiastic passer-by followed the crime suspect from behind, until reaching Long Ping Estate where he notified the police. The police rushed to arrest the suspect and took him in. The two victims were taken to hospital by ambulance. [繼上月26日大角嘴有精神病患者在街頭「無差別」持刀追斬女途人後，元朗再發生「翻版」血案。一名有傷人前科的精神病患者，昨在街頭用鎅刀襲擊兩名女途人後，若無其事棄刀步行離去；幸有熱心途人尾隨跟蹤疑兇至朗屏邨報警，由警員趕至拘捕疑兇帶署，兩名傷者由救護車送院。] (#72)

From the outset of the opening paragraph of this *Ming Pao* report, the reported crime is linked to a similar recent crime, marked linguistically by the expressions "following on from," "again," and "copycat." These point to the recurring nature of such crime in Hong Kong. The opening paragraph names the present perpetrator and his predecessor through their illness, with the former described as having "a record of assault." This implicitly links the apparent increasing frequency of crimes of this type in Hong Kong to people with a severe mental illness who, seemingly, repeatedly commit violent assault. Both perpetrators are agents of actions that connote fear and violence, namely, "wielding," "chasing," "knifing," and "attacked." The opening paragraph calls attention to the randomness of their actions through its use of the adverb "indiscriminately," accentuated by the use of quotation marks. This gives credence to the description in appearing to cite the words of a witness or a police source. The opening paragraph also engenders senses of randomness and familiarity, by describing the victims as "passers-by"; and by identifying the locations of the attacks as "on the street" and in named localities. Other *Ming Pao* crime reports similarly call attention to the unpredictability of crime committed by people with a severe mental illness at this upper level of the news text superstructural hierarchy, through their frequent use of qualifiers such as "sudden" [突], "for no reason" [無故], "not known" [不相識], "opportunistic" [乘機], "out of control" [失控], and "mad" [狂]. The opening paragraph of this crime report additionally points to the callousness of the mentally ill perpetrator, by noting that he walked away from a violent "bloody crime" "as if nothing had happened." Such callousness, by extension, could be shared by many people with a severe mental illness, given that they can be "copycats." Definitively introduced by the positive adverb "fortunately," the opening paragraph immediately contrasts this callousness with the warmth and gallantry of a mentally well bystander, namely, a man who follows the perpetrator and notifies the police. As such, the now legalistically named "crime suspect" is subject to the subordinating acts of being pursued (by an everyday male bystander) and detained (by the police).

24. On 5 December last year <u>in Chiaohsi, Yilan</u>, a <u>man by the name of Chou</u> sent a <u>menacing</u> text signed "<u>Cheng Chieh Fan Club</u>," <u>threatening Dun-Hua Elementary School in Taipei, You-Chang Elementary School in Kaohsiung, and Chang-Hua Girls Senior High School</u>. He <u>warned</u>, "<u>this motherfucker</u> has put <u>explosive devices</u> in <u>hidden</u> locations at these schools, and is preparing to properly <u>blow everyone to smithereens, slither-slather</u>. There's no point notifying the police." He also criticised that <u>Wei-Chuan sold tainted cooking oil scot-free</u>, with KP [the mayor of Taipei] saying that the law is just there for reference. He wants to "<u>marshal up</u> thousands to <u>rob and loot</u>." The Taipei district court yesterday sentenced Mr Chou to 4 months in prison for the crime of <u>public menace, allowing appeal</u>. Mr Chou argued in court that he had repeatedly reported a neighbour's illegal construction, but to no avail. Believing that the law is dead, he devised a plan to use <u>threatening</u> means to make his case, but did not actually act or plan to let off a bomb. The judge determined that Mr Chou <u>jeopardised public order and safety</u>, just because <u>a very trivial matter</u> was not able to be resolved. He should not have done so. However, considering he has no previous convictions and <u>suffers from depression</u>, he was <u>given a light sentence</u>. [宜蘭礁溪周姓男子去年12月5度[日]寄電子恐嚇信署名「鄭傑後援會」，恐嚇台北市敦化國小、高雄市右昌國小、彰化女中，揚言「林北已在學校隱密處放置炸彈爆裂物，準備好好大炸得皮開肉綻、唏哩嘩啦，報警也沒用」，還批評連味全賣黑心油都可無罪，柯P也說法律僅供參考，他要「集結萬人來搶劫」；台北地院昨依恐嚇公眾罪，判周男4月徒刑。可上訴。周男到案辯稱，一再檢舉鄰居的違章建築，卻長期沒有解決，他認為法律已死，才起意以恐嚇手法表達訴求，但並無實際放炸彈的

行為與計畫，法官認定周男只因細故未能得到解決，即危害公眾秩序安全，實屬不該，考量他無前科且患憂鬱症，未予重判。] (#127)

Like Example 23, this opening paragraph of a *Liberty Times* crime report familiarises the crime by clearly identifying where it was to take place. The opening paragraph further heightens the attendant threat to the general "public" by specifying that the crime was to take place in named schools. This means that its victims would have been innocent local schoolchildren. The report calls attention to this threat at this upper level of the news text super-structural hierarchy through its repeated use of expressions such as "menace," "threaten," and "jeopardise." It further positions the legalistically named per-petrator as the agent of ominous and frightening verbs, such as "warn," "mar-shal," "rob," "loot," and "blow to smithereens, slither-slather." The opening paragraph gives voice to the perpetrator, but what he says is very disturbing. He vulgarly calls himself "this motherfucker," and nonsensically links his proposed attack, which terrifyingly uses "hidden explosive devices," to the duplicitous selling of fake cooking oil with impunity. Most disturbingly, it only takes "a very trivial matter" to trigger the attack. Once again, the opening paragraph of the report points to the recurring nature of such crime in the local commu-nity. This stems, by implication, from its naming of the notorious mentally ill mass murderer "Cheng Chieh," of whom the perpetrator is a "fan." Cheng ran-domly stabbed several passengers to death on a Taipei subway in 2014. Another *Liberty Times* crime report pointedly names Wang Ching-Yu [王景玉] in its opening paragraph. Wang randomly decapitated a young girl on a Taipei street in 2016. The opening paragraph contrasts the cold-heartedness of the mentally ill perpetrator with the graciousness of his sentencing judge, who "allows" him "to appeal" and "gives him a light sentence." One clear difference between this opening paragraph and its *Ming Pao* counterpart is the latter's naming of the perpetrator by way of his severe mental illness from the very outset, while the former delays mention of severe mental illness to the very last sentence.

The opening paragraphs of a number of other *Liberty Times* crime reports draw on gender in different ways to their *Ming Pao* counterparts. The former commonly point out ways in which people with a severe mental illness trans-gress gender norms in Chinese culture. Descriptions in the opening paragraph may include a woman's personal status as divorced or living in a de-facto relationship; or as being a single mother, prostitute, pornographic film actor, or estranged from her parents. These states of being contravene normative femininity in Chinese culture, where women are expected to be virtuous, get married, and dutifully take care of elders (Croll 1995; Guo 2010). Descriptions of a man similarly may include his personal status as unemployed, an alco-holic, an illicit drug user, or a "weirdo" [怪客]. These states of being contra-vene normative masculinity in Chinese culture, where men are expected to be honourable, righteous, and gainfully employed (Louie 2002, 2015; Lu 2012; Ramsay 2016). As a result, these reports bear out the long-standing stigmatic construction of people with a mental illness in Chinese culture as transgressive and unproductive. They are unable to fulfil their gender roles.

The opening paragraphs of other *Liberty Times* crime reports also differ from their *Ming Pao* counterparts in prioritising the voice of perpetrators with a severe mental illness. By contrast, the *Ming Pao* and *People's Daily* counterparts prioritise the voice of those in authority or family members. Any empowerment that the perpetrators may gain from this, however, is diminished by the alarming or farcical statements that they make (see selected Examples 25 and 26).

25. After Criminal Suspect You was restrained, <u>he actually said that he likes to kill people. He also said, "Cockroaches are life too. I want to save them!"</u> [游嫌被制住後，竟稱自己喜歡殺人，又說：「蟑螂也是生命，我要救牠們！」] (#239)
26. The police rushed to arrest the person. They asked, "Why didn't you run away?" <u>Miss Chang amazingly replied, "Because I have no experience [in robbing jewellery stores]."</u> [警方趕到逮人，警方問：「怎不逃跑？」張女神回：「沒有經驗」。] (#256)

Thus, while the opening paragraphs of a number of *Liberty Times* crime reports afford voice to perpetrators with a severe mental illness, the articulation of positive and productive claims remains the province of those in authority. Moreover, the opening paragraphs of these reports direct greater attention to victims with a severe mental illness, in line with the actual experience of crime for those with the illness, yet concurrently diminish their agency. This is because the opening paragraphs deny them a voice, while casting them as passive recipients of other people's transgressions; or as agents of distinctly negative actions (see selected Examples 27 and 28).

27. 2 years living constantly <u>under the shadow of being drugged and sexually assaulted</u>, she consequently developed depression. [2年來一直活在遭受餵毒性侵的陰影下，因此罹患憂鬱症。] (#201)
28. Miss Liao, who has depression, <u>swallowed 6 sleeping pills</u>. Mr Tsai then <u>took advantage of</u> her drowsiness and <u>abused</u> her by <u>setting fire to</u> her hair, face, and thigh, amongst other places. [有憂鬱症的廖女吞了6顆安眠藥，蔡男竟趁廖女昏睡之際，用火燒廖女頭髮、臉部、大腿等處凌虐。] (#284)

At this upper level of the news text superstructural hierarchy, most *Liberty Times* crime reports displace blame for a victim's severe mental illness, in an empowering way, onto the crime that is perpetrated against them, as indicated by Example 27's use of the causal marker "consequently." Reports seldom displace blame for the crime onto their illness, as Example 28 may imply through its use of the sequential marker "then."

The opening paragraph of the *People's Daily* crime reports, which, of course, are very few in number, is highly legalistic and institutional in tone. Frequent use of nominalisation and passive voice emphasise institutional agency over individual agency (see selected Example 29 below). The openings of sentences name or allude to state institutions, such as the prosecutor's office, forensic psychiatry, the courts, and the law. Example 29 specifically makes mention of the "nation," which does not occur in the *Ming Pao* and *Liberty Times* counterparts. Doing so affirms that the upcoming court sentence will be valid and sound, because it carries the backing of the state.

29. Several days ago, <u>the prosecutor's office</u> approved <u>the arrest</u> of <u>the suspect</u> in the Sichuan Normal University <u>murder case, a certain</u> Mr Teng, <u>on suspicion of premeditated homicide.</u> Previously, the results of <u>the psychiatric assessment</u> of this <u>certain</u> Mr Teng had showed that he suffers from depression. He <u>was judged</u> as having <u>partial criminal responsibility</u> for his actions on the day of the crime. <u>In accordance with the relevant provisions of our nation's criminal law,</u> there can be some <u>leniency in sentencing.</u> [日前，四川师范大学凶杀案嫌疑人滕某，因涉嫌故意杀人罪被检察机关批准逮捕。此前，滕某的精神鉴定结果显示其患抑郁症，案发当天行为被评定为部分刑事责任能力。依照我国刑法的相关规定，可以从轻、减轻处罚。] (#4)

In sum, the opening paragraphs of the news reports on crime where severe mental illness is implicated in the three Chinese-language newspapers discursively align to a greater degree than their headlines do. At this upper level of the news text superstructural hierarchy, the reports from all three newspapers legalistically fortify the link between severe mental illness and crime. They further call attention to the random nature of such crime. Problematic reporting of this kind also characterises Western reporting of mental illness (see Chapter 1 section on news media reporting of mental illness in the West), which, in like manner, gives greater attention to "hetero-aggressive acts" directed at others, rather than to "auto-aggressive ones" directed at self (Rukavina, Nawka, Brborović et al. 2012, p. 1141). The crime reports in the three Chinese-language newspapers contrast the apparent danger posed by people with a severe mental illness with the goodness and gallantry of mentally well citizens, usually men. This only marginalises and disempowers people with a mental illness to a greater degree.

The opening paragraphs of these news reports in all three newspapers also prioritise the voice of people in authority. What they say institutionally validates widely held stigmatic attitudes towards and beliefs about people with a severe mental illness in culturally Chinese communities, namely that they are helpless, unproductive, erratic, dangerous, and best removed from everyday society (see Chapter 1 section on Chinese discourse studies on mental illness). As such, they do not challenge and, so, potentially transform, readers' "habits of mind" in relation to severe mental illness, that is, people's entrenched ways of thinking about and responding to the illness, in nuanced, humanising, and inclusive ways (Gibson & Jacobson 2018, p. 187).

There, however, are some differences and nuances in the ways in which the opening paragraphs of these news reports construct severe mental illness in detrimental ways. The *Ming Pao* reports continue to name people, in a reductive way, through their illness, as they did in their headlines. The *Liberty Times* and *People's Daily* counterparts do not, instead assigning legalistic and institutional labels that, nonetheless, are equally dehumanising. The *Ming Pao* reports further marginalise severe mental illness, by proximally linking it to family poverty, intellectual disability, and social taboos. The *Liberty Times* counterparts similarly link it to socially denigrated states of being, but, more notably, to those that violate traditional gender norms in Chinese culture. The *People's Daily* reports, meanwhile, appear to use the detrimental construction of severe mental illness for a political purpose. They do so by concomitantly calling attention to the party's and state's deep concern about, and well thought-out responses to, crime where severe mental illness is implicated. They further point out how this pressing social issue bears out one of the nation's leading contemporary political tenets, namely "rule by law" [依法治国]. This tenet positively marks out the stable, constituted governance of the post-1978 Open Door reform period on the mainland from the tumultuous rule of the preceding Cultural Revolution period (1966–1976).

Beyond their opening paragraphs, the crime reports from all three newspapers continue to display discursive practices that characterise their headlines and opening paragraphs. The *Ming Pao* and *People's Daily* reports are legalistic in tone, giving vocal privilege to police, judges, or lawyers, rather than to those with a severe mental illness; and naming perpetrators with such illness as "the defendant" [被告] or "a certain" Mr/s such and such [某]. The *Ming Pao* reports give greater attention to court proceedings as a consequence of a crime, since most of them are rudimentary summaries of published court case documents. The *Ming Pao* and *People's Daily* reports both construct crime in ways that blur the distinction between law and biomedicine. They do so by chronicling perpetrators' erstwhile diagnoses of severe mental illness > their recent intentional stopping of medication > the subsequent resurfacing of their psychiatric symptomatology > their progression to often aggressive, antisocial behaviour > their committing of a crime. They also back up medical claims by reference to a "psychiatric report" [精神科報告], or a "previous record of severe mental illness" [有精神病前科]. This authoritative report or record, in an orthodox biomedical way, names a psychiatric diagnosis, and recommends hospitalisation and medical treatment of those with a severe mental illness. Judges recontextually incorporate this language into their court verdicts. As a result, the hospitalisation and medical treatment of those with a severe mental illness become legally mandated. This legitimises their forensic removal from everyday society into prison-like psychiatric facilities, such as *Ankang* on the mainland and Siu Lam Psychiatric Centre in Hong

Kong (Angermeyer & Schulze 2001; Blood, Putnis, & Pirkis 2002; Clement & Foster 2008).

The *Ming Pao* crime reports additionally provide greater background on people with a severe mental illness, at this lower level of the news text superstructural hierarchy. They detail people's medical histories, family circumstances, residential settings, and socioeconomic status. Rather than sympathetically contextualising the lives of these people, the reports further cast them in a negative light. People suffer frequent relapses of their severe mental illness. They do not work; need constant "care" [照顧] and "follow-up" [跟進] from government agencies; permanently live with their families, or in inadequately staffed halfway houses; and have their children taken away into state care. The reports never cast them, in an empowering way, as active agents of change.

By contrast, the *Liberty Times* crime reports give greater attention to the medical progress of victims of crime; financial compensation that courts award them; family atonement for the perpetrator's actions; and reactions of the community or authorities to the crime (see selected Examples 30 and 31).

30. Overnight, at the Yuping police station, <u>the parents of criminal suspect Kuo constantly apologised to the owners of the damaged vehicles</u>. They left their contact details and <u>promised to take responsibility for compensation</u>. [前晚郭嫌父母在育平所內不斷向受害車主道歉，並留下聯絡資料，承諾會負責賠償。] (#111)

31. <u>Mr Lu's aunty was taken to hospital for emergency treatment, but died from her injuries</u>. When brought back to the police station, Mr Lu said, "Someone told me to kill my father as well," which <u>completely shocked the police officers</u>. [呂男姑姑送醫急救不治，呂男被帶回警局時說：「有人叫我連爸爸一起殺」，讓員警震驚不已。] (#150)

The reports do not set out the medical histories of those with a severe mental illness, or point out their unflattering life circumstances. This casts them in a more positive light than their *Ming Pao* counterparts do. The *Liberty Times* reports on *victims* of crime, nevertheless, tend to be longer than those on perpetrators of crime. This may be because the crimes against people with a severe mental illness are often quite salacious and, so, more likely to retain the readers' attention.

The reporting in the lower levels of the news text superstructural hierarchy in all three newspapers continues to subordinate the voice of people with a severe mental illness. People in authority speak on their behalf. What they say disempowers those with a severe mental illness, by consigning them to the care, management, and control of health professionals and legislators. A *Ming Pao* and a *People's Daily* crime report are exceptions. The former reports exclusively on Thomas Mair, a British man with a severe mental illness, who recently had murdered a U.K. member of parliament. It concludes by quoting Mair's younger brother, who claims that "[Mair] is not violent and not obsessed with politics and [...] had received help for his long-standing severe mental illness" [哥哥不暴力，也不熱中政治... 他患精神病多年，有接受協助] (#34). This report is about a foreigner (from a Hong Kong reader's perspective), which places some distance between the brother's positive appraisal of the mentally ill Mair and local stigmatic attitudes towards and beliefs about severe mental illness. Moreover, the brother's reported comments appear at the lowest level of the news text superstructural hierarchy. They also include the descriptors "<u>not</u> violent" and "<u>not</u> obsessed," which, while negated, implicitly call attention to two manifestly undesirable traits that stereotypically characterise people with a severe mental illness in Chinese culture. In like manner, the *People's Daily* crime report quotes a past teacher of a male sex offender, who has a severe mental illness. The teacher claims that the offender was a "filial" [很孝順] and "well-behaved student" [一位品行良好的学生] at school, adding that, with "treatment" [治疗], he could "be a scholar who contributes to society" [做一位对社会有贡献的学者] (#21). These comments call attention to desired states of being in contemporary mainland Chinese society. They also call attention to the redemptive power of the mainland Chinese state and its affiliates, in bringing about these states of being. By corollary, they imply that people with a severe mental illness who shun medical treatment can never contribute to society in a productive capacity.

This ongoing silence of those with a severe mental illness means that other people, mostly those in authority, tell their story. The stories that they tell align, in a disempowering way, with a biomedical-cum-institutional narrative that espouses support, management, and control of those with a severe mental illness. The ongoing silence of those with a severe mental illness also amplifies their social and cultural other-ness. Readers will readily construct people whose voices they do not hear in line with prevailing audible narratives. The audible narrative about severe mental illness in Chinese societies is decidedly stigmatic (see Chapter 1 section on Chinese discourse studies on mental illness). As a result, the readers' own deep-seated attitudes towards and beliefs about people with the illness, that is, their "habits of mind" (Gibson & Jacobson 2018, p. 187), will remain unchallenged and unchanged.

In sum, the lower levels of the news text superstructural hierarchy of the crime reports from all three newspaper continue to prioritise the voice of people in authority. This adds credibility to claims made in the reports. The authoritative voice in the *Ming Pao* and *People's Daily* reports further blurs the distinction between law and biomedicine. As a result, state authorities can use orthodox biomedical rationales and protocols to correctively manage and control those with a severe mental illness. This often means their removal from everyday society, in line with long-standing stigmatic attitudes and beliefs in culturally Chinese communities. Blurring the distinction between law and biomedicine in this way also allows the mainland Chinese authorities to showcase their rational, yet redemptive, responses to a pressing social issue. These responses clearly align with the state's key political tenets of rule by law [依法治国], and of maintaining social harmony and social stability on the mainland. The *Ming Pao* crime reports further disclose intrusive, unflattering, private information about people with a severe mental illness. This devalues their personhood. The *Liberty Times* counterparts, on the other hand, document more charitable aspects of their lives, if they are victims of crime. These reports also attribute the victims' severe mental illness to the crime perpetrated against them. By contrast, their *Ming Pao* and *People's Daily* counterparts implicitly attribute the crime to the victims' illness.

Suicide in present-day greater China

Suicide is not a crime in most countries of the world. This includes the regions that make up greater China. Nevertheless, analysis of the reports on suicide where severe mental illness is at issue sits alongside analysis of those on crime where the illness is implicated, due to the emergent discursive commonalities between these two thematic categories of reports. That is to say, the three Chinese-language newspapers report on suicide and crime of this type in very similar ways.

The act of suicide differs across Chinese and Western societies in that, in the former, it can bring honour in death (Maggs 2012; Pearson & Liu 2002; Pearson, Phillips, He et al. 2002; Wu 2010). This is because Chinese cultural norms and scripts construct suicide as a powerful "act of resistance when" people are "wronged" by their loved ones or the broader society (Wu 2010, p. 53). Through death, people who face intractable, shameful, troubled circumstances, such as domestic conflict or external dispute, can find "justice," "gain face," and restore their "human dignity" (Wu 2010, pp. 6, 13,131). As such, "suicide is usually seen as a social problem [and] not a medical one in China" (Wu 2010, p. 5).

This greater socialisation of suicide is borne out by Wu's (2010) claim that severe mental illness causes more than 90% of completed (fatal) suicides in the West, yet only 63% of completed suicides in mainland China. Bi, Tong, Liu et al. (2010) and Tong, Phillips, and Conner (2016) cite similar figures for both suicide attempts and completed suicides in mainland China and the West. Wu (2010) points to a possible explanation for this pronounced cross-cultural difference in suicide aetiology. Long-standing stigmatic attitudes and beliefs in mainland China deem that people with severe mental illness are "non-persons" (Wu 2010, p. 94). As such, their suicides "do not count" (Wu 2010, p. 94). This may skew aetiological explanations for suicide away from severe mental illness and onto more positively regarded phenomena.

Traditionally, the gender distribution for suicide in mainland China has differed markedly from that in the West, with many more women than men suiciding in the former (Wu 2010). The numbers of women committing suicide in mainland China, however, has plummeted in recent times. Zhang (2019) states that "[t]he most marked decrease has been observed in young women in rural areas younger than 35 years, whose suicide rate appears to have decreased by as much as 90%" (p. 1533). Zhang (2019) explains that this stems from contemporary rural women's greater social freedom, independence, and self-confidence as migrant workers in urban centres; their lack of immediate access to the agricultural pesticides that rural dwellers commonly use to commit suicide on impulse; the greater valuing of women in mainland China, due to the proportional surplus of marriage-age men arising from the decades-long one-child policy; improved mental health support in schools; and state control over media reporting on suicide. As a result, since 2011, the gender distribution for suicide in mainland China has come to resemble that in the West (Wang, Chan, & Yip 2014; Zhang, Sun, Liu et al. 2014). The Global Health Data Exchange (GHDx) database maintained by the Institute for Health Metrics and Evaluation at the University of Washington, U.S.A., calculates a suicide rate for men and women in mainland China in 2017 of around eleven per 100,000 and 7.5 per 100,000, respectively (GHDx 2018). Men also are overrepresented in suicide statistics across the West and in most nations across the globe (Galasiński 2013, 2017; Sun & Zhang 2017; Wang, Chan, & Yip 2014).

GHDx (2018); Wang, Chan, and Yip (2014); Zhang, Sun, Liu et al. (2014); and Zhang (2019) put the overall suicide rate in contemporary mainland China at around eight per 100,000 people. This is a substantial decrease compared to the overall suicide rate at the turn of the twenty-first century (Tong, Phillips, & Conner 2016). Wang, Chan, and Yip (2014) caution, however, that the rate would approach ten per 100,000 people if unreported suicides were included. Such a rate would still be lower than the World Health Organization's global estimate for 2012 of 11.4 suicides per 100,000 people (Sun & Zhang 2017). It would also be considerably lower than GHDx's estimate for Australia in 2017, namely, around thirteen suicides per 100,000 people (GHDx 2018). Sun and Zhang (2017); Tong, Phillips, and Conner (2016); Wang, Chan, and Yip (2014); and Zhang, Sun, Liu et al. (2014) add that the rate of suicide in rural and remote areas of mainland China remains higher than its urban areas. Moreover, the rate of suicide for elderly people in mainland China is higher than that for younger age groups (Wang, Chan, & Yip 2014; Zhang, Sun, Liu et al. 2014).

Overall rates of suicide are somewhat higher in Taiwan and Hong Kong. Taiwan's Ministry of Health and Welfare reports that the rate for Taiwan in 2016 was 12.3 suicides per 100,000 people (Ministry of Health & Welfare 2017). This was down from 15.3 suicides per 100,000 people in 2013 (Lung, Liao, Wu et al. 2017). GHDx, however, puts the rate in 2017 at more than eighteen suicides per 100,000 people, suggesting a return to levels much higher than those in mainland China and Australia (GHDx 2018). Hsu, Chang, Lee et al. (2015) estimate that the rate of suicide in Hong Kong is around fourteen per 100,000 people for young men and eight per 100,000 people for young women, rising up to forty per 100,000 people for elderly men and 21 per 100,000 people for elderly women. They add that men accounted for 62% of suicides in Hong Kong between 2005 and 2010. The corresponding figure for Taiwan between 1999 and 2007 was quite similar, with men accounting for 68.4% of suicides (Chang, Sterne, Wheeler et al. 2011). GHDx confirms a similar gender distribution pattern for suicide in Taiwan in 2017 (GHDx 2018). This overrepresentation of men in suicide statistics in Taiwan extends across its urban, rural, and remote areas (Chang, Sterne, Wheeler et al. 2011). Chang, Sterne, Wheeler et al. (2011) add that the rate of suicide in Taiwan, like that in mainland China, is higher in its rural and remote areas than in its urban areas. Yet, unlike mainland China and Hong Kong, young people, namely, Aboriginal men, are overrepresented in suicide statistics in Taiwan (Chang, Sterne, Wheeler et al. 2011).

Analyses by Bi, Tong, Liu et al. (2010); Cheng (1995); and Sun and Zhang (2017) suggest that these distributional patterns in suicide across present-day greater China hold whether or not there is comorbid severe mental illness.

Suicide reports

Ming Pao and *Liberty Times* report on suicide where severe mental illness is at issue much more commonly than the *People's Daily* does. This points to the political sensitivity of the topic for the mainland Chinese authorities (Zhang 2019). The relative frequencies with which *Ming Pao* and *Liberty Times* report on the topic are very similar, at around one in every six to seven reports on severe mental illness. All three newspapers report on suicide by women with a severe mental illness more often than they report on suicide by men with this illness. This is despite the fact that men proportionally more often commit suicide across greater China. This apparent underreporting of suicide by men with a severe mental illness in all three newspapers supports findings by Chen, Yip, Tsai et al. (2012, p. 144) that newspapers in Taiwan "underreport mental illness as a reason for suicide in men," yet readily link it to suicide in women. It may be that linking suicide to severe mental illness, an intensely stigmatised state of being in Chinese culture, is less problematic in the case of women, due to their traditionally subordinate status in Chinese culture. Alternatively, being a woman may sensationalise the act of suicide, especially when it is violent, given that gruesome acts by women are often deemed more culturally transgressive and, so, attention-grabbing, than those by men (Drakeley 2007; Pohlman 2015).

All of the *Liberty Times* reports and nearly all of their *Ming Pao* counterparts appear in the local news section of the newspaper (see Appendices 2 and 3). Here, they are more likely to be read by the readers. The *Liberty Times* reports cluster across December to March, while their *Ming Pao* counterparts cluster in January and March (see Appendices 2 and 3). There is no clear explanation for these clusters, with reports describing different incidents of suicide as well as different methods for committing suicide. The *Liberty Times* reports solely deal with adult suicide, while their *Ming Pao* and *People's Daily* counterparts more frequently deal with youth suicide. This is despite the fact that suicide is more common amongst the elderly in Hong Kong and mainland China. While all the *Liberty Times* and *People's Daily* reports point to depression as a cause of suicide, only a small number of *Ming Pao* reports do (see Appendices 1–3). They, instead, mostly point to generic severe mental illness as a cause of suicide; or expressly deny that severe mental illness had any bearing on a reported suicide. Such denials may preserve honour in suicide. Having severe mental illness renders suicide ignominious, since it reduces the status of the suicide victim to that of a "non-person" (Guo 2016, p. 196). As such, her or his suicide does not "count" (Wu 2010, p. 94). At the same time, the denials antithetically call attention to the causal link between severe mental illness and suicide. This is because they imply that readers would instinctively make such a link. There are only three *People's Daily* suicide reports published over the extended twelve-month period of analysis (see Appendix 1).

None of the headlines of the *Ming Pao* and *People's Daily* reports on suicide where severe mental illness is at issue make any mention of severe mental illness. Less than one-third of the headlines of their *Liberty Times* counterparts do so. The *Liberty Times* headlines that mention the illness (always depression) do so in an opening clause; or reductively name the suicide victims by way of their illness (see selected Examples 32 and 33).

32. <u>Suffers From Depression</u> – Woman Hairdresser <u>Jumps Off Building To Her Death</u> [罹患憂鬱症 女美髮師墜樓亡] (#131)
33. Daxi Charred Corpse Shock – <u>Depressed Woman Self-Immolates</u> [大溪赫見焦屍 憂鬱婦自焚] (#151)

It is noteworthy that headlines like these name the illness at this highest level of the news text superstructural hierarchy, since very few headlines of *Liberty Times* reports from across all the thematic categories do so. In naming the illness, the headlines not only link it to suicide, but to sensationally violent suicide, such as "jumping off a building" and "self-immolation." They concomitantly explicitly or implicitly call attention to loss of life, through use of lexis such as "death" and "corpse." Some headlines further contrast the disturbing acts of those who suicide with the heroic and principled actions of rescuers or family members (see selected Example 34).

34. Depressed Man Tries To Lie On Railway Tracks – Quick-Witted Police Officer Placates Him, Drags Him Back [鬱男欲臥軌 機智警安撫拉回] (#165)

These discursive features of the headlines of the suicide reports are reminiscent of those of the headlines of the crime reports (see this chapter's section on crime reports). As such, the headlines similarly make full use of the disturbingly sensational and so, commercial, value of a violent act. Suicide, accordingly, is cast as an ignominious act and not an honourable one, as tradition may have it. This occurs whether or not a headline expressly names severe mental illness. Despite this sensational construction of suicide, a small number of headlines of *Ming Pao* reports cite academic and professional advice about suicide where severe mental illness is at issue (see selected Example 35).

35. Cheung Hing-Yee: Changing Opinion About Suicide Since 90s: Why Do We Have To Be Happy? [張馨儀：90年代至今自殺輿論變遷：為什麼不得不快樂？] (#55)

The headlines of *People's Daily* reports on suicide where severe mental illness is at issue, while few in overall number, are similarly didactic (see selected Example 36).

36. *People's Daily*: Do Not Ignore Child's Anxiety [人民日報：別忽視孩子的焦慮] (#11)

Both Examples 35 and 36, in an institutional way, name those in authority from the outset of the headline. This gives credence to the ensuing opinion and advice. They are heralded, once again in typically institutional ways, by a question posed by the expert, or a directive in the form of an imperative clause. This citing of authoritative opinion and advice at the highest level of the news text superstructural hierarchy may stem from the *Ming Pao* and *People's Daily* suicide reports' focus on youth suicide. Such reports would be especially confronting to culturally Chinese communities that traditionally view suicide as an honourable act carried out by shamed or socially conflicted *adults*. This may call for authoritative opinion and advice on why young people would wish to suicide and how to deal with this emerging social calamity. Such opinion and advice is absent from the *Liberty Times* suicide reports, which, by contrast, focus on adult suicide, for which a cogent cultural explanation already exists.

In sum, the headlines of the suicide reports in all three newspapers vividly construct suicide as a violent act, reminiscent of a crime. As a result, they cast suicide as sensational social wrongdoing rather than a culturally honourable act of social rectitude or resistance. Sensationalising suicide in this way goes against the World Health Organization's "media reporting recommendations" for suicide (Chu, Zhang, Cheng et al. 2018, p. 454). The headlines of the suicide reports in the three newspapers also make no mention of severe mental illness. This, too, goes against WHO recommendations for reporting on suicide, which state that any such reporting should openly "[a]cknowledge the link between suicide and mental disorders like depression" (Chu, Zhang, Cheng et al. 2018, p. 454). Chu, Zhang, Cheng et al. (2018, p. 459) find that only 8% of suicide reports in mainland Chinese newspapers acknowledge this link, while around 52.6–76.4% of comparative Australian reports do. The intense cultural stigma against severe mental illness in Chinese societies may explain this stark difference across geographical settings.

The headlines draw much greater attention to youth suicide in severe mental illness in *Ming Pao* and the *People's Daily*, than in *Liberty Times*. The former further complement their focus on youth suicide, in typically institutional ways, by citing authoritative opinion and advice. By contrast, *Liberty Times*, which solely reports on adult suicide in severe mental illness, lacks such complementary coverage. Prevailing cultural scripts surrounding suicide may explain this.

Two *Liberty Times* suicide reports have lead paragraphs that state an anti-suicide message and list the contact details for a suicide prevention hotline. Doing so is line with WHO recommendations for reporting on suicide (Chu, Zhang, Cheng et al. 2018). The remaining *Liberty Times* reports and all the *Ming Pao* counterparts that solely report on an act of suicide launch directly into the description of the main event, namely, the act of suicide. Their descriptions are routinely graphic, confronting, and linked to death (see selected Examples 37 and 38).

37. A 19-year-old pregnant girl, who was due to give birth at the end of this month, yesterday <u>climbed out of a window of a friend's apartment at Shep Kip Mei Estate and jumped off</u>. The suspected cause is complications from prenatal depression. <u>She broke through a van's windscreen, dropping down into its cabin, seriously injured. She died</u> in hospital. After investigating, the police had no doubt that this was a case of someone <u>falling from a great height</u>. They temporarily handed it over to the major crime unit of the Sham Shui Po police district for follow-up. The 19-year-old female victim, named Ng, was <u>unconscious with multiple fractures to her head and body</u> when discovered. <u>She died</u> in hospital. <u>The foetus that she had carried for more than 9 months also died.</u> [一名預產期為本月底的19歲孕婦疑因產前抑鬱症困擾，昨日在親友石硤尾邨寓所攀窗墮樓，壓穿一輛客貨車擋風玻璃跌入車廂重傷，送院不治。警方調查後認為無可疑，列作有人從高處墮下案處理，暫交由深水埗警區重案組跟進。女事主姓吳，19歲，被發現時頭部及身體多處骨折昏迷，送院不治，其所懷9個多月胎兒亦死亡。] (#41)

38. Midday yesterday, a 54-year-old woman by the name of Yang was found <u>wedged in a 20cm-wide crevice between a certain hotel building and the building next door on West Min-Sheng Road in North Town. She</u> was taken to the hospital emergency department, but <u>died</u>. Early investigation by the police shows that Ms. Yang booked into a room on the 9th floor of the hotel on the 7th. She had disclosed to friends in recent days her intention to commit suicide, a result of suffering from depression and bone cancer. Police are trying to ascertain the cause of <u>death</u>. [54歲楊姓女子，昨日中午被發現卡在北市民生西路某飯店大樓與隔壁棟大樓20公分寬的夾縫中，經送醫急救仍不治；警方初步調查，楊女7日投宿該飯店9樓，因罹患憂鬱症和骨癌，近日才向親友吐露輕生念頭，警方正追查死因。] (#155)

These two main event paragraphs are typical of the suicide reports in their respective newspapers. They describe the act of suicide as one akin to crime. They recount where a suicide took place; name the person who commits suicide; describe the method of suicide; and document the police rescue response or investigation into the fatality. Police involvement, therefore, is discursively conspicuous. However, the voice of the victims, for example, from the time leading up to their suicide, is rarely heard. The reports also characteristically feminise suicide, even though men more commonly commit suicide in Hong Kong and Taiwan.

The *Ming Pao* report (Example 37) draws greater attention to the gender of the suicide victim, pointing out from the very outset that she was late-stage pregnant. It does not personally name her until much later in the paragraph. Moreover, it repeatedly alludes to her gender, by causally linking her pregnancy to her severe mental illness and, in turn, her suicide; and by declaring that her late-stage foetus had died. It further identifies her fatal "prenatal depression," even though formal medical confirmation was yet to be received. By contrast, the *Liberty Times* report (Example 38) identifies the woman suicide victim by her personal name from the very outset of the paragraph, albeit in a legalistic way that is reminiscent of crime reports. Other *Liberty Times* suicide reports similarly label victims as "the deceased" [死者] or the "corpse" [屍]. Although the *Liberty Times* report causally links the victim's suicide to her severe mental illness, as the *Ming Pao* report does, it does not persistently gender her suicide. It further makes this causal link between suicide and severe mental illness much later in the paragraph.

Just under half of the *Ming Pao* suicide reports carry denials of severe mental illness in the case that they report on. There are no such denials in their *Liberty Times* counterparts. The denials still call attention to severe mental illness, by implying that people would generally associate it with suicide (Tang & Bie 2015). Its absence, therefore, becomes newsworthy. The denials also may preserve the sense of honour that can surround an act of suicide in Chinese culture (Maggs 2012; Pearson & Liu 2002; Pearson, Phillips, He et al. 2002; Wu 2010). By suiciding, social transgressors can remove the stain and shame that they have brought upon their families. Being labelled mentally ill, however, would erase such honour in suicide, due to the intense stigma against severe mental illness in Chinese culture, which genetically extends to one's family members (Dikötter 1998; Ramsay 2008, 2013; Tang & Bie 2015). The family members of a person with a severe mental illness would remain socially tainted and shamed, regardless of whether the person is alive or dead.

While small in number, the *People's Daily* suicide reports rather differently describe suicide in an orthodox biomedical way. They do so at this upper level of the news text superstructural hierarchy, by including illustrative personal anecdotes about suicide, using cause-and-effect rhetoric, and pointing to authoritative statistics. In this way, they set up a social problem, namely suicide, for which a manageable solution grounded in biomedicine is set out in the remainder of the report. A solution of this type sits comfortably within the state's ambit.

In sum, the main event of the reports on suicide where severe mental illness is at issue differs in part across the three newspapers. The *Ming Pao* and *Liberty Times* reports continue to construct suicide as a graphically violent act, reminiscent of crime. Their *People's Daily* counterparts, however, cast it more as a medical problem. This would make the problem more politically palatable and manageable. While the reports in all three newspapers mostly deal with women victims, counter to statistical trends for gender in suicide, those in *Ming Pao* appear to make greater use of gender for voyeuristic sensational impact. A number of *Ming Pao* reports also stand out due to their denials of severe mental illness in individual cases of suicide. Such denials may retain a vestige of cultural honour in the act of suicide, by removing the potentially stigmatic effect of comorbid severe mental illness.

Nearly all of the *Ming Pao* suicide reports continue on with details about the circumstances leading up to a suicide, in the lower levels of their news text superstructural hierarchy. By contrast, less than half of their *Liberty Times* counterparts do so. The longer *Ming Pao* reports may stem from their making full voyeuristic use of suicide, in particular, that by women, for sensational value. In detailing the circumstances that led up to a suicide, these reports implicitly or explicitly point to a cause. The *Ming Pao* reports equally blame severe mental illness alone; prevailing social structures and ideologies that ignore individual diversity; family crises or ignorance; and the victims themselves for not seeking psychiatric help earlier on, not adhering to family planning, or not being aware of the many opportunities that a chosen career presents. Their *Liberty Times* counterparts, by contrast, do not directly blame wider society, families, or the victims themselves, instead pointing to severe mental illness alone, chronic physical illness, heredity, work pressures, and earthquakes. The *People's Daily* suicide reports, while very few in number, also continue on with details about the circumstances leading up to a suicide in the lower levels of their news text superstructural hierarchy. They, however, uniformly blame suicide on family crises and ignorance. This removes the wider society, and the infallible state that governs it, from any culpability. By corollary, responsibility to solve this problem ultimately rests with the family, under the didactic command and tutelage of "the nation" [我国] or "motherland" [祖国] (see selected Examples 39 and 40).

39. To make children receive proper protection and prevent "infection" with harmful feelings, <u>adults should take responsibility and use a positive attitude and actions in life to set an example for children.</u> [让孩子们受到应有的保护，防止不良情绪的"感染"，成年人应该担起责任，以积极正面的人生态度和行动，给孩子们树立榜样。] (#11)

40. Thus, <u>parents must care about and pay attention to a child's mood changes, and especially must take extra care of a child during a rebellious phase,</u> in order to avoid a young life being destroyed in the most beautiful

of years. [因此，家长要关心和重视孩子的情绪变化，特别是要多加呵护叛逆期的孩子，以免年轻的生命毁灭在最美的年华。] (#23)

This shifting of responsibility for a social problem onto families and, so, away from the unerring state is also evident in the *People's Daily* crime reports.

In sum, the suicide reports in all three Chinese-language newspapers tend to relegate the immediate causes of suicide to the lower levels of the news text superstructural hierarchy, or not mention them at all. The *Ming Pao* reports on occasion assign broader communal blame for suicide, while their *Liberty Times* and *People's Daily* counterparts do not. As such, the *Liberty Times* reports are less culturally affronting to readers, while their *People's Daily* counterparts preserve the meritorious standing of the state and the society it governs.

Severe mental illness as crime and social wrongdoing

Newspapers face a crucial choice when reporting on severe mental illness, especially when crime and social wrongdoing such as ignominious suicide are at issue. They can choose to luridly sensationalise these events, attracting the attention of readers and, so, increasing commercial sales. Alternatively, they can take the opportunity to counter the prevailing stigma against severe mental illness in society by reporting on such events in considered and measured ways that bear out the everyday experience of the illness and point to how society can positively contribute to improvements in this experience. The discourse analysis in this chapter shows that reporting on crime and social wrongdoing where severe mental illness is at issue in the three Chinese-language newspapers, similar to that characterising Western reporting, tends to sensationalise the experience of the illness, but to varying degrees and for differing purposes.

Ming Pao and *Liberty Times* give disproportionate attention to confronting, extraordinary events where severe mental illness is at issue, namely, violent crime perpetrated by those with the illness, and gruesome suicides by them. This highly negative portrayal of the experience of severe mental illness usually appears in commonly read sections of the newspapers. The opposite is true of the *People's Daily*, which appears to eschew such reporting, most likely due to political imperatives (Zhang 2019). These may include the need to avoid reporting on issues that could call into question the state's paramount concern for maintaining social harmony, social stability, and the rule of law on the mainland (Brady 2008, 2009; Cao 2014; Choy 2016; Sandby-Thomas 2014).

While disproportionately reporting on crime and suicide where severe mental illness is at issue, the analysis shows that *Liberty Times* does so in a way that is less stigmatising and disempowering than *Ming Pao*. The former gives greater attention to people with a severe mental illness who are victims of crime, as well as to adults with the illness who commit suicide. This is more in line with the reality of these tragic experiences for those with the illness.

In doing so, the newspaper provides greater insight into the experience of women with a severe mental illness. It also commonly specifies the diagnostic name of the illness in question, in most cases depression. Doing so helps avoid a wholesale stigmatic dismissal of those with a severe mental illness as an undifferentiated "other," completely at odds with "normal" people (Georgaca & Bilić 2007, p. 175).

Liberty Times also is comparatively less stigmatising in rarely making mention of severe mention illness in the headlines of its crime reports and suicide reports. This means that no immediate association between the illness and violent crime or suicide is made at the highest levels of the news text superstructural hierarchy. Newspaper readers, therefore, are less likely to gain and retain such associations, especially if they merely browse headlines, as many do (van Dijk 1988a, 1988b). In addition, the newspaper does not name people with a severe mental illness by way of their illness in the ensuing news story. This avoids essentialising them in a way that diminishes their humanity, as their *Ming Pao* counterparts commonly do. Moreover, the *Liberty Times* reports often displace blame for severe mental illness onto external social factors and forces, while many *Ming Pao* counterparts, by implication, blame those with the illness. Doing so only further stigmatises them. The schematic structure of the *Liberty Times* reports is also less legalistic in form than their *Ming Pao* counterparts. This potentially reduces discernible overtones of criminality.

The lexis of the crime reports and suicide reports in all three newspapers, nevertheless, is highly legalistic, linking severe mental illness to criminality. This further stigmatises and dehumanises those with the illness. They are reported on in ways that common criminals are. They also lack any substantive voice. Instead, their experience of severe mental illness is told by those in authority, usually the police, judges, lawyers, and health professionals. Their authoritative accounts are not only replete with the lexis of law and biomedicine, but also recontextually obscure the boundaries between these two disciplines. Doing so readily recasts the removal of those with a severe mental illness away from everyday society as a just and humane act.

All three newspapers also similarly gender their reports on crime and suicide in ways that disempower women with a severe mental illness. The women are passive and often acted upon by men. They lack voice and transgress gender norms. This is even so in the *Liberty Times* reports, which otherwise stigmatise and disempower less regularly than their *Ming Pao* and *People's Daily* counterparts do. Women in all three newspapers commit suicide more often than men do, contrary to the statistical reality across greater China. Their suicides also are sensationally violent and ignominious, despite the potential for the act to be honourable in Chinese culture. This likely is because the comorbid presence of severe mental illness necessarily renders the act ignoble, due to the long-standing intense stigma against the illness in Chinese culture. Sensationalising suicide in this way goes against WHO recommendations for reporting on suicide (Chu, Zhang, Cheng et al. 2018).

Ming Pao, therefore, regularly reports on crime and suicide where severe mental illness is at issue in ways that adversely sensationalise the illness. This finding is common to Western reporting on the illness (see the Chapter 1 section on news media reporting of mental illness in the West). *Liberty Times*, by contrast, is just as likely to report on such crime and suicide in ways that adversely sensationalise severe mental illness, as to do so in ways that magnanimously humanise and normalise it. The *People's Daily* crime reports and suicide reports, on the other hand, stand out due to their paucity in number, and their use of crime and suicide where severe mental illness is at issue for political purpose. They consistently direct blame for such crime and suicide away from the unerring state. At the same time, they actively point out positive responses and achievements by the state. These responses and achievements are rationally grounded in science, and benefit the whole nation. Chapter 5 further examines this co-opting of severe mental illness for political or activist gain. Beforehand, the next chapter evaluates the extent to which, how, and why the three Chinese-language newspapers narrate people's life stories of severe mental illness.

Notes

1 All translations in this and subsequent chapters are the author's, unless otherwise indicated. Translations tend to be "faithful" to the source text, in order to maintain, as much is possible, the linguistic features of the source text.

2 # denotes the number of the news article, as listed in Appendices 1, 2, and 3.

3 In order to maintain a degree of idiomaticity while retaining the basic linguistic structure of the expression, the book translates *jingshenbinghuanzhe* [精神病患者] as "mental illness sufferer," rather than the semantically more precise, but structurally more cumbersome, "severe mental illness sufferer." However, *jingshenbing* [精神病] is still translated as the structurally uncumbersome and semantically more precise "severe mental illness." The Chapter 1 section on the analysis of Chinese-language print media reports on mental illness outlines the rationale for using the qualifier severe.

References

Angermeyer, M. C., & Schulze, B. (2001). Reinforcing stereotypes: How the focus on forensic cases in news reporting may influence public attitudes towards the mentally ill. *International Journal of Law and Psychiatry*, 24(4), 469–486.

BBC Monitoring Asia Pacific (2016, 12 September). Hong Kong media facing credibility crisis, survey shows. London, UK. https://search.proquest.com/docview/1818284777?accountid=14723.

Bi, B., Tong, J., Liu, L., Wei, S., Li, H., Hou, J., Tan, S., Chen, X., Chen, W., Jia, X., Liu, Y., Dong, G., Qin, X., & Phillips, M. R. (2010). Comparison of patients with and without mental disorders treated for suicide attempts in the emergency departments of four general hospitals in Shenyang, China. *General Hospital Psychiatry, 32*(5), 549–555.

Blood, R. W., Putnis, P., & Pirkis, J. (2002). Mental-illness news as violence: A news frame analysis of the reporting and portrayal of mental health and illness in Australian media. *Australian Journal of Communication, 29*(2), 59–82.

Brady, A. (2008). *Marketing dictatorship: Propaganda and thought work in contemporary China.* Lanham, MD: Rowman & Littlefield.

Brady, A. (2009). Mass persuasion as a means of legitimation and China's popular authoritarianism. *American Behavioral Scientist, 53*(3), 434–457.

Burnett, A., Mattern, J. L., Herakova, L. L., Kahl, D. H. Jr., Tobola, C., & Bornsen. S. E. (2009). Communicating/muting date rape: A co-cultural theoretical analysis of communication factors related to rape culture on a college campus. *Journal of Applied Communication Research, 37*(4), 465–485.

Candlin, C. N. (2001). Medical discourse as professional and institutional action: Challenges to teaching and researching languages for special purposes. In M. Bax & C. J. Zwart (Eds.), *Reflections on language and language learning: in honour of Arthur van Essen* (pp. 185–207). Amsterdam: John Benjamins.

Cao, Q. (2014). Introduction: Legitimisation, resistance and discursive struggles in contemporary China. In Q. Cao, H. Tian, & P. A. Chilton (Eds.), *Discourse, politics and media in contemporary China* (p1–24). Amsterdam: John Benjamins.

Cashman, E. L., & Thomas. S. D. M. (2017). Does mental illness impact the incidence of crime and victimisation among young people? *Psychiatry, Psychology and Law, 24*(1), 33–46.

Chan, O., & Chow, K. K. W. (2014). Assessment and determinants of aggression in a forensic psychiatric institution in Hong Kong, China. *Psychiatry Research, 22*(1–2), 623–630.

Chan, S. K. W., Ching, E. Y. N., Lam, K. S. C., So, H., Hui, C. L. M., Lee, E. H. M., Chang, W. C., & Chen, E. Y. H. (2017). Newspaper coverage of mental illness in Hong Kong between 2002 and 2012: Impact of introduction of a new Chinese name of psychosis. *Early Intervention in Psychiatry*, 11(4), 342–344.

Chang, S. S., Sterne, J. A. C., Wheeler, B. W., Lu, T. H., Lin, J. J., & Gunnell, D. (2011). Geography of suicide in Taiwan: Spatial patterning and socioeconomic correlates. *Health Place, 17*(2), 641–650.

Chen, Y., Yip, P. S. F., Tsai, C., & Fan, H. (2012). Media representation of gender patterns of suicide in Taiwan. *Crisis: The Journal of Crisis Intervention and Suicide Prevention, 33*(3), 144–150.

Cheng, A. T. A. (1995. Mental illness and suicide: A case-control study in East Taiwan. *Archives of General Psychiatry, 52*(7), 594–603.

Choy, H. Y. F. (2016). Introduction: Disease and discourse. In H. Y. F. Choy (Ed.), *Discourses of disease: Writing illness, the mind and the body in modern China* (pp. 1–15). Leiden: Brill.

Chu, X., Zhang, X., Cheng, P., Schwebel, D. C., & Hu, G. (2018). Assessing the use of media reporting recommendations by the World Health Organization in suicide news published in the most influential media sources in China, 2003–2015. *International Journal of Environmental Research and Public Health, 15*(3), 451–462.

Clement, S., & Foster, N. (2008). Newspaper reporting on schizophrenia: A content analysis of five national newspapers at two time points. *Schizophrenia Research, 98*(1), 178–183.

Corbin, J. M., & Strauss, A. L. (2008). *Basics of qualitative research: Techniques and procedures for developing grounded theory* (3rd ed.). Thousand Oaks, CA: SAGE.

Cowan, G. (2000). Women's hostility toward women and rape and sexual harassment myths. *Violence Against Women, 6*(3), 238–246.

Croll, E. (1995). *Changing identities of Chinese women: Rhetoric, experience and self perception in twentieth century China.* Hong Kong: Hong Kong University Press.

Dikötter, F. (1998). *Imperfect conceptions: Medical knowledge, birth defects and eugenics in China.* London: Hurst & Co.

Drakeley, S. (2007). Lubang Buaya: Myth, misogyny and massacre. *Nebula, 4*(4), 11–35.

Every-Palmer, S., Brink, J., Chern, T. P., Choi, W. K., Hern-Yee, J. G., Green, B., Heffernan, E., Johnson, S. B., Kachaeva, M., Shiina, A., Walker, D., Wu, K., Wang, X., & Mellsop, G. (2014). Review of psychiatric services to mentally disordered offenders around the Pacific Rim. *Asia Pacific Psychiatry, 6*(1), 1–17.

Fraser, J. (1999). The discourse of official texts and how it can impede public service translators. *Journal of Multilingual and Multicultural Development, 20*(3), 194–208.

Galasiński, D. (2008). *Men's discourses of depression.* London: Palgrave Macmillan.

Galasiński, D. (2013). *Fathers, fatherhood and mental illness: A discourse analysis of rejection.* London: Palgrave Macmillan.

Galasiński, D. (2017). *Discourses of men's suicide notes: A qualitative analysis.* New York: Bloomsbury Academic.

Georgaca, E., & Bilić, B. (2007. Representations of "mental illness" in Serbian newspapers: A critical discourse analysis. *Qualitative Research in Psychology, 4*(1), 167–186.

Gibson, C., & Jacobson, T. (2018). Habits of mind in an uncertain information world. *Reference and User Services Quarterly, 57*(3), 183–192.

Global Health Data Exchange. (2018). http://ghdx.healthdata.org/gbd-results-tool.

Guo, J. (2016. *Stigma: An ethnography of mental illness and HIV/AIDS in China.* Hackensack, NJ: World Century.

Guo, Y. (2010). China's celebrity mothers: Female virtues, patriotism and social harmony. In L. Edwards, & E. Jeffreys (Eds.), *Celebrity in China* (pp. 45–66). Hong Kong: Hong Kong University Press.

Harper, D. J. (1995). Discourse analysis and "mental health." *Journal of Mental Health, 4*(4), 347–357.

Harper, S. (2009). *Madness, power and the media: Class, gender and race in popular representations of mental distress.* Basingstoke, UK: Palgrave Macmillan.

Hong Kong Correctional Services. (2018). Siu Lam Psychiatric Centre. www.csd.gov.hk/english/facility/facility_ind/ins_nt_slpc.html.

Hsu, C. C., Sheu, C. J., Liu, S. I., Sun, Y. W., Wu, S. I., & Lin, Y. (2009). Crime victimization of persons with severe mental illness in Taiwan. *Australasian Psychiatry, 43*(5), 460–466.

Hsu, C. Y., Chang, S. S., Lee, E. S. T., & Yip, P. S. F. (2015). Geography of suicide in Hong Kong: Spatial patterning, and socioeconomic correlates and inequalities. *Social Science and Medicine, 130*(2015), 190–203.

Iedema, R. (1997). The language of administration: Organizing human activity in formal institutions. In F. Christie, & J. R. Martin (Eds.), *Genre and institutions: Social processes in the workplace and school* (pp. 73–118). London: Cassell.

Judicial Yuan of the Republic of China. (2018). Law and Regulations Retrieving System. http://jirs.judicial.gov.tw/index.htm.

Kesic, D., Ducat, L. V., & Thomas, S. D. (2012). Using force: Australian newspaper depictions of contacts between the police and persons experiencing mental illness. *Australian Psychologist, 47*(4), 213–223.

Kleinman, A., Yan, Y., Jun, J., Lee, S., Zhang, E., Pan, T., Wu, F., & Guo, J. (2011). *Deep China: The moral life of the person: What anthropology and psychiatry tell us about China today.* Berkeley, CA: University of California Press.

Knifton, L., & Quinn, N. (2008). Media, mental health and discrimination: A frame of reference for understanding reporting trends. *International Journal of Mental Health Promotion, 10*(1), 23–31.

Li, G., Gutheil, T. G., & Hu, Z. (2016). Comparative study of forensic psychiatric system between China and America. *International Journal of Law and Psychiatry, 47*(2016), 164–170.

Louie, K. (2002). *Theorising Chinese masculinity: Society and gender in China.* Cambridge: Cambridge University Press.

Louie, K. (2015). *Chinese masculinities in a globalizing world.* New York: Routledge.

Lu, Y. (2012). *Heroic masculinity and male homosociality in* Three Kingdoms *and* Le Morte Darthur [Doctoral dissertation, University of Queensland].

Lung, F. W., Liao, S. C., Wu, C. Y., & Lee, M. B. (2017). The effectiveness of suicide prevention programmes: Urban and gender disparity in age-specific suicide rates in a Taiwanese population. *Public Health, 147*(2017), 136–143.

Maggs, E. (2012). *A cultural analysis of suicide in the Chinese classical novels* Romance of the Three Kingdoms *and* Dream of Red Mansion [BA Honours dissertation, University of Queensland].

Mann, S. K. F., & Chong, B. B. W. (2016). How stigma from the public and significant others affects self-perception in people with mental illness in Hong Kong: A qualitative study. *Hong Kong Journal of Social Work, 50*(1/2), 3–25.

Ministry of Health and Welfare. (2017). *Taiwan health and welfare report 2017.* Ministry of Health and Welfare, R.O.C. (Taiwan).

Mishler, E. G. (1984). *The discourse of medicine: Dialectics of medical interviews.* Norwood: Ablex.

Olstead, R. (2002). Contesting the text: Canadian media depictions of the conflation of mental illness and criminality. *Sociology of Health and Illness, 24*(5), 621–643.

Pearson, V. (1996). The Chinese equation in mental health policy and practice. *International Journal of Law and Psychiatry, 19*(3/4), 437–458.

Pearson, V., & Liu, M. (2002). Ling's death: An ethnography of a Chinese woman's suicide. *Suicide and Life-Threatening Behaviour, 32*(4), 347–358.

Pearson, V., Phillips, M. R., He, F., & Ji, H. (2002). Attempted suicide among young rural women in the People's Republic of China: Possibilities for prevention. *Suicide and Life-Threatening Behaviour, 32*(4), 359–369.

Phillips, M., Chen, H., Diesfeld, K., Xie, B., Cheng, H., Mellsop, G., & Liu, X. (2013). China's new mental health law: Reframing involuntary treatment. *American Journal of Psychiatry, 170*(6), 588–591.

Pohlman, A. (2015). *Women, sexual violence and the Indonesian killings of 1965–1966.* London: Routledge.

Ramsay, G. (2008). *Shaping minds: A discourse analysis of Chinese-language community mental health literature.* Amsterdam: John Benjamins.

Ramsay, G. (2013). *Mental illness, dementia and family in China.* London: Routledge.

Ramsay, G. (2016). *Chinese stories of drug addiction: Beyond the opium dens.* New York: Routledge.

Richardson, J. E. (2007). *Analysing newspapers: An approach from Critical Discourse Analysis.* New York: Palgrave Macmillan.

Rukavina, T. V., Nawka, A., Brborović, O., Jovanović, N., Kuzman, M. R., Nawková, L., Bednárová, B., Zŭchová, S., Hrodková, M., & Lattova, Z. (2012). Development of the PICMIN (picture of mental illness in newspapers): Instrument to assess mental illness stigma in print media. *Social Psychiatry and Psychiatric Epidemiology, 47*(7), 1131–1144.

Sandby-Thomas, P. (2014). "Stability overwhelms everything": Analysing the legitimating effect of the stability discourse since 1989. In Q. Cao, H. Tian, & P. A. Chilton (Eds.), *Discourse, politics and media in contemporary China* (pp. 47–76). Amsterdam: John Benjamins.

Shi-xu. (2014). *Chinese discourse studies.* Hampshire, UK: Palgrave Macmillan.

Shi-xu. (2015). Towards a cultural methodology of human communication research: A Chinese example. In L. Tsung & W. Wang (Eds.), *Contemporary Chinese discourse and social practice in China* (pp. 45–58). Amsterdam: John Benjamins.

Sun, L., & Zhang, J. (2017). Gender differences among medically serious suicide attempters aged 15–54 years in rural China. *Psychiatry Research, 252*(2017), 57–62.

Tang, L., & Bie, B. (2015). Narratives about mental illnesses in China: The voices of Generation Y. *Health Communication, 31*(2), 171–181.

Tong, Y., Phillips, M. R., & Conner, K. R. (2016). DSM-IV Axis II personality disorders and suicide and attempted suicide in China. *The British Journal of Psychiatry, 209*(4), 319–326.

Topiwala, A., Wang, X., & Fazel, S. (2012). Chinese forensic psychiatry and its wider implications. *Journal of Forensic Psychiatry and Psychology, 23*(1), 1–6.

van Dijk, T. A. (1988a). *News as discourse.* Hillsdale, NJ: Lawrence Erlbaum.

van Dijk, T. A. (1988b). *News analysis: Case studies of international and national news in the press.* Hillsdale, NJ: Lawrence Erlbaum.

van Dijk, T. A. (2000). *Ideology: A multidisciplinary approach.* Thousand Oaks, CA: SAGE.

van Dijk, T. A. (2014). Discourse, cognition, society. In J. Angermuller, D. Maingueneau, & R. Wodak (Eds.), *Discourse Studies reader: Main currents in theory and analysis* (p388–399). Amsterdam: John Benjamins.

van Dijk, T. A. (2015). Critical Discourse Analysis. In D. Tannen, H. E. Hamilton, & D. Schiffrin (Eds.), *The handbook of discourse analysis* (p466–485). Malden, MA: Wiley Blackwell.

Varshney, M., Mahapatra, A., Krishnan, V., Gupta, R., & Deb, K. S. (2016). Violence and mental illness: What is the true story? *Journal of Epidemiology and Community Health, 70*(3), 223–225.

Wahl, O., Wood, A., & Richards, R. (2002). Newspaper coverage of mental illness: Is it changing? *Psychiatric Rehabilitation Skills, 6*(1), 9–31.

Wang, C. W., Chan, C. L. W., & Yip, P. S. F. (2014). Suicide rates in China from 2002 to 2011: An update. *Social Psychiatry and Psychiatric Epidemiology, 49*(6), 929–941.

Wang, W., & Liu, Y. (2016). Discussing mental illness in Chinese social media: The impact of influential sources on stigmatization and support among their followers. *Health Communication, 31*(3), 355–363.

Wodak, R. (1996). *Disorders of discourse.* New York: Longman.

Wu, F. (2010). *Suicide and justice: A Chinese perspective.* New York: Routledge.

Xu, X., Li, X. M., Xu, D., & Wang, W. (2017). Psychiatric and mental health nursing in China: Past, present and future. *Archives of Psychiatric Nursing, 31*(5), 470–476.

Xue, L., Shi, Y. W., Knoll, J., & Zhao, H. (2015). Chinese forensic psychiatry: History, development and challenges. *Journal of Forensic Science and Medicine, 1*(1), 61–67.

Yang, T. W., Yu, J. M., & Pan, C. H. (2017). Analysis of concordance between conclusions of forensic psychiatric evaluation and court decisions after 2005 Criminal Code Amendment in a Taiwan psychiatric hospital. *International Journal of Law and Psychiatry, 54*(2017), 148–154.

Zhang, J. (2019). Suicide reduction in China. *American Journal of Public Health, 109*(11), 1533–1534.

Zhang, J., Sun, L., Liu, Y., & Zhang, J. (2014). The change in suicide rates between 2002 and 2011 in China. *Suicide and Life-Threatening Behavior*, 44(5), 560–568.

4 Life stories of severe mental illness

Chapter 3 shows that the contemporary Chinese-language news reports on crime and suicide where severe mental illness is at issue discursively endorse the dominant cultural narrative operating across greater China. As such, they diminish and disempower those with the illness in ways that bear out long-standing stigmatic attitudes and beliefs in culturally Chinese communities. This chapter analyses news reports that narrate people's life stories of severe mental illness. This includes the life stories of people who have the illness, as well as those of family members who care for them. Chapter 5 subsequently deals with accounts of health professionals who provide specialist care for those with a severe mental illness.

Chapter 2 shows that the *Ming Pao* and *Liberty Times* reports that narrate people's life stories of severe mental illness proportionally trail those on crime and suicide where the illness is at issue. Reports that narrate people's life stories account for 26–30% of all reports in the two newspapers, while their crime reports and suicide reports account for 40–53%. These two newspapers, seemingly, prioritise reporting on more sensational happenings in severe mental illness. Not only do their reports thematically neglect the personal experience of severe mental illness, but when they do report on it they disproportionately prioritise the life stories of well-known celebrities. Their life stories appear to be more newsworthy than those of everyday people. This disregard for the everyday personal experience of severe mental illness is even starker in the *People's Daily*. Across an extended twelve-month time frame of analysis, the newspaper solely reports on the celebrity experience of severe mental illness and never reports on that of everyday people.

This chapter identifies the ways in which the reports in the three leading Chinese-language newspapers narrate people's life stories of severe mental illness. It compares and contrasts how they recount the life stories of both celebrities and everyday people. It examines the extent to which the narrative voices of celebrities and everyday people humanise and empower those with a severe mental illness in mainland China, Hong Kong, and Taiwan. It also considers the reasons for any differences across these three geographical regions. The analysis proceeds as in Chapter 3.

The voice of the lifeworld

Medical humanities research over the past few decades has pointed out the potential benefits of giving greater voice to those who suffer from an illness. Doing so can counter the dominance of the orthodox voice of health professionals and their affiliated institutions when it comes to description and discussion of an illness experience. This orthodox doctor-centred biomedical voice, as opposed to one that is more client-centred and mutually reflective, is highly logical, rational, uniform, and prescriptive (Dixon-Woods 2001; Fleischman 2003; Ramsay 2008; Roberts & Sarangi 1999; Samovar & Porter 2001; Sarangi 1998). It tends to "devalue emotion and intuition as sources of knowledge" (Macionis, quoted in Samovar & Porter 2001, p. 63), and "prize rationality, objectivity, empirical evidence, and the scientific method" (Samovar & Porter 2001, p. 63). By contrast, the "lifeworld" voice of those who suffer from an illness is more nuanced (Mishler 1984, p. 104). It gives greater, more personal attention to "social context and experiences rather than solely relying on signs, symptoms, and demonstrable pathologies" (Dixon-Woods 2001, p. 1418).

Giving greater voice to those who suffer from an illness, therefore, can contribute to a fuller understanding of the day-to-day experience of an illness: one which emphasises and, so, normalises, diversity and difference (Ainsworth-Vaughn 2003; Bhui & Bhugra 2002; Fleischman 2003; Harper 1995, 1996; MacDonald 1998). The ways in which these people narrate their life stories of illness provide insight into how they make temporal and causal sense of it in their lives, as well as how they draw on it to cultivate or refashion emergent notions of self or identity (Hunt 2000; Hurwitz 2004; Hydén 1997; Hydén & Brockmeier 2008; Hydén & Örulv 2009; Ramsay 2010, 2013; Riessman 2004). Their narration necessarily involves the use of language, which, consequently, has discursive import and impact on what it means to have an illness in a cultural setting (Galasiński 2008, 2013; Garden 2010; Kleinman 1988; Lafrance 2007; Lupton 2003; Mishler 1984; Ramsay 2010, 2013; Sontag 1989).

Newspapers are one medium where these life stories can be told. In the Chinese-language newspapers under study, such stories may counterbalance the disproportionate, detrimental attention to crime and social wrongdoing where severe mental illness is at issue (*Ming Pao* + *Liberty Times*); or the disproportionate, disempowering attention to current medical findings about, and government policy on, the illness (*People's Daily*). However, the extent to which narrating life stories provides such a counterbalance depends on who narrates them and in what way. This requires deeper discourse-level analysis.

Celebrity reports

Reports on the celebrity experience of severe mental illness proportionally equal or outnumber those on the experience of everyday people in all three newspapers (see Appendices 1–3). The *Liberty Times* reports narrowly focus on two male vocalists from two boy bands that are popular in Taiwan, namely, Ting Ting [廷廷] from "Magic Power" [MP魔幻力量]; and Jet [易桀齊] from "51." Both men suffer from depression. The focus on these men contributes in part to the seventeen *Liberty Times* reports on male celebrities' experience of severe mental illness well outnumbering the four reports on the experience of women celebrities. If calculating by individual celebrity, these figures reduce to seven different men and four different women. Either way, reports on male celebrities dominate *Liberty Times* numerically. By contrast, reports on male celebrities are in the minority in *Ming Pao* and the *People's Daily*.

The *Ming Pao* and *Liberty Times* celebrity reports deal almost exclusively with depression (see Appendices 2 and 3). Their *People's Daily* counterparts more often deal with generic severe mental illness (see Appendix 1). Publication of the *People's Daily* and *Ming Pao* celebrity reports does not cluster in any one month (see Appendices 1 and 2). Publication of their *Liberty Times* counterparts, however, clusters in January, February, and April of 2016 (see Appendix 3). This is due to their ongoing reporting of issues related to Ting Ting's and Jet's depression. Publication of the celebrity reports in all three newspapers unsurprisingly clusters in their entertainment sections (see Appendices 1–3).

The sensational and, so, commercial value of reporting on celebrities is borne out in the headlines across all three Chinese-language newspapers. They typically name the celebrities or their celebrity affiliation, such as their music band's name or film's title, at the outset of the headline (see selected Examples 1–3).

1. Joey Wong Shares Recent Photos Celebrating 49th Birthday – Got Depression? Become Nun? Has Illegitimate Daughter? Rough Lot For Goddess [王祖贤晒近照庆生49岁 得抑郁症？出家？有私生女？看女神坎坷命运] (#12)
2. Rain Lau: Luckily Scared Of Death – Suffers Depression, Contemplates Suicide [劉玉翠：幸自己驚死 患抑鬱症曾想輕生] (#94)
3. Irene Chen – Depression, Hair Loss, Failed Marriage – Regrets Being Artist [陳艾琳憂鬱鬼剃頭 婚姻失敗悔當藝人] (#164)

Examples 1–3 report on women celebrities and make explicit mention of their severe mental illness at this highest level of the news text superstructural hierarchy. None of these headlines set the women celebrities as agents of unequivocally positive, honourable, empowering actions. This is typical of the headlines of the celebrity reports in all three newspapers. Example 1 from the *People's Daily* topicalises the name of the woman celebrity and then poses three questions about her in the succeeding clause, namely, whether she "has depression"; whether she "has become a Buddhist nun"; and whether she "has an illegitimate daughter." In this way, she is proximally linked to life circumstances and events that many mainland Chinese readers would find decidedly unpleasant, curious, or shameful. In like manner, Examples 2 and 3 from *Ming Pao* and *Liberty Times*, respectively, call attention to decidedly negative life circumstances and events, at this highest level of the news text superstructural hierarchy.

By contrast, only some of the headlines of the celebrity reports that deal with male celebrities do so. Male celebrities more commonly are agents of positive, honourable, empowering actions, unless they suffer from schizophrenia (see selected Examples 4 and 5).

4. Boy Band "51" <u>Goes Past</u> Depression – <u>Engrossed In</u> Jade Design [男團51走過憂鬱 醉心翡翠設計] (#173)
5. "Star Wars" Child Star <u>Sent To Hospital</u> With Schizophrenia [《星戰》童星思覺失調送院] (#56)

Example 4 from *Liberty Times* awards members of the well-known all-male music band positive agency in successfully overcoming their depression and conscientiously committing to other valued vocational pursuits. In this way, they make productive contributions to society, in line with normative masculinity in Chinese culture (Louie 2002, 2015). By contrast, Example 5 from *Ming Pao* diminishes the agency of the well-known (male) film star, who is removed from everyday society as a result of his schizophrenia, denoted by the neologism *sijueshitiao*. The headline grammatically conceals who sent him to hospital, by way of the passive voice. This maintains attention on the newsworthy film star. The removal of people with schizophrenia from everyday society aligns with stigmatic Chinese cultural expectations (Guo 2016; Kleinman, Yan, Jun et al. 2011; Ramsay 2013). Other headlines describe male celebrities' severe mental illness as "tragic" [慘]. This never occurs for women celebrities at this highest level of the news text superstructural hierarchy (see selected Examples 1–3).

The celebrity reports in all three Chinese-language newspapers lack summary lead paragraphs. Their reporting of the main event of the news story designates celebrities by way of their personal names or stage names from the outset of the paragraph. This verifies their newsworthiness. The reporting of the main event also identifies their illness, but for seemingly different discursive purposes across the three newspapers. Illness naming has distinct biomedical airs in the *People's Daily* celebrity reports. This is because their reporting clearly states or implies that illness labels are assigned by health professionals:

• "severe mental illness sufferer Joker Xue" [重度精神病患者薛之谦] (#1).
• "only later on, after seeing the doctor, did she realise that she was suffering from severe depression" [后来看了医生，她才知道自己患上了严重的抑郁症] (#19).
• "diagnosed with mild schizophrenia and depression" [被诊断为轻度精神分裂和抑郁症] (#28).

The *Ming Pao* and *Liberty Times* celebrity reports, however, appear to name an illness as part of a broader narrative strategy to inspire readers through personal testimony. At this upper level of the news text superstructural hierarchy, these testimonies give greater voice to those with a severe mental illness, here, the celebrity, as they temporally contrast the adverse challenges they faced when they were acutely symptomatic with their active triumphs and principled realisations in recovery (see selected Examples 6–9).

6. In fact, as early as 2013, when Wentworth Miller "came out," he revealed that he had suffered the hardship of depression since he was a young man. But this time, he told of another low ebb in his life: "2010 was the lowest point of my adult life" [...] Yet, since then he has sought out the meaning behind all of this. For him, these [paparazzi] pictures [of him when he was very unwell] represent "strength, recovery, and forgiveness – forgiveness of oneself and others." [其實早於2013年當溫禾夫米勒「出櫃」時，已自爆從他少年時代開始已受抑鬱症之苦，只是今次他再細訴另一段人生低潮，「2010年，是我成年後人生的最低潮」[...] 但之後他會尋找背後的意義，對他來說這些照片代表了「力量、復元及原諒，原諒自己及其他人。」] (#61)

7. She stated: "I have gone through depression and the process is very difficult" [...] She said: "This song, hopefully, will encourage everyone to face up to problems of the mind. Don't try to avoid them. Bravely face up to the issue of depression." [她表示：「我經歷過抑鬱症，過程好艱難」[...] 她說：「今次的歌曲是希望鼓勵大家面對心靈的問題，不要去逃避，勇敢面對抑鬱症的問題。」] (#95)

8. Eli Hsieh (centre) has left behind the shadow of depression. He not only has released a new album, but also sang solo last night at a venue jam-packed with more than 600 fans. [謝震廷(中)，走出憂鬱症陰影後，不僅推出新專輯，前晚還舉辦個唱，現場擠滿600多位歌迷。] (#181)

9. Roger Yang has a history of depression lasting 7 years. On top of that, his grandfather and father passed away in succession these past few years. The day after he finished writing his new song "The End," he truly tried to "end it" when he attempted suicide by taking drugs. Fortunately, he was saved. But this made him muse over his painful experience. He deeply feels that if he abandons his mother and wife, his grandfather and father in heaven would not be pleased. Having realised this, his current motto is "live in the moment" – he hopes to live every day nicely. He hopes that his own model of what not to do can serve as a reverse example and bring positive thinking to all. [楊培安有憂鬱症病史長達7年，加上這幾年爺爺、爸爸接連過世，寫完新歌《了斷》的隔一天，真的自我「了斷」仰藥輕生，所幸獲救，但這也讓他痛定思痛，深覺若拋下母親和妻子，在天上的爺爺和爸爸也不會開心，領悟之後，他現在的座右銘是「活在當下」，希望好好的過每一天。 他希望自身的錯誤示範，可以是個反面教材，帶給大家正面思考。] (#191)

A male and female celebrity with depression speak of their negative experiences when ill in Examples 6 and 7 from *Ming Pao*. Both subsequently positively reinterpret their experiences to inspire others: morally through encouraging outright "forgiveness," and didactically through calling for "strength," "recovery," and courage. In like manner, Examples 8 and 9 from *Liberty Times* inspirationally point to the positive achievements of two male celebrities following their reportedly negative experiences of depression. These achievements are gendered in line with normative masculinity in Chinese culture, through the men's overt displays of productivity and vocational success; patriarchal honour and filial piety; and social benevolence and altruism (Louie 2002, 2015). All these examples maintain attention on the celebrities with depression, through their grammatical agency as regular subjects of clauses. Example 9 additionally conceals the agency of the others who had saved Roger Yang, through its use of the passive voice. By contrast, their *People's Daily* counterparts do not bestow agency on the celebrities with a severe mental illness in these ways. For them, severe mental illness is not experiential but a diagnostic label assigned by doctors.

Nevertheless, the *Ming Pao* and *Liberty Times* reports on celebrities with schizophrenia also deny them agency at this upper level of the news text superstructural hierarchy. Others, such as a family member or a health professional, commonly speak on their behalf (see selected Example 10 below). In addition, those in authority remove them from everyday society into prison-like institutions, as Chinese cultural stigma would dictate (see selected Example 10).

10. Jake Lloyd <u>was transferred by the authorities to a psychiatric hospital</u> in recent times. What <u>his mother, Lisa, has divulged</u> confirms that he is suffering from schizophrenia: <u>"punishment cannot solve his problem – the only way out is through treatment." She also stated</u> that she had visited her son in hospital last week, and was pleased to see that his condition had taken a turn for the better. However, <u>the doctor said</u> that he has no timetable for discharge for the time being. [直至最近被當局移送到精神病院，據他的母親Lisa透露，積萊特證實患上思覺失調，「懲罰並不能解決他的問題，接受治療才是出路」。她又表示，上周曾入院探望兒子，喜見病情已有好轉，不過，醫生說他暫時未有出院的時間表。] (#56)

Despite the *Liberty Times* celebrity reports appearing to inspire readers through personal testimony about success and achievement in severe mental illness, at the same time, they regularly document adverse, often scandalous, celebrity behaviours and actions. This is not the case in their *People's Daily* and *Ming Pao* counterparts, at this upper level of the news text superstructural hierarchy. Sensational behaviours and actions of the ill celebrities include sexual indiscretion, substance abuse, petty theft, imprecation, suicide attempts, dangerous driving, bullying, separation, and divorce (see selected Examples 11 and 12).

11. "MP Magic Power" has again suffered explosive allegations. It surprisingly has been revealed that lead singer, Ting Ting, who temporarily <u>left the band</u> after suffering from severe depression, <u>groped a female actor</u> in an idol drama. [「MP魔幻力量」又遭爆料，暫離團的主唱廷廷深受憂鬱症所苦，竟爆沾上偶像劇的女演員。](#116)
12. Debby Wang <u>disappeared from the limelight for all of last year</u>. Rumour has it that she, who has bipolar disorder, also is suffering from depression. The fuse was her <u>falling out with her bestie of many years</u>, Carolyn Chen. When she was interviewed by the media not long ago, she suddenly <u>got extremely fired up</u> on hearing the words "Carolyn Chen," <u>ferociously alleging: "That stinking X tore into me over a no-hoper of a man!"</u> [楊琪去年消失螢光幕1年，傳出有躁鬱症的她又罹患憂鬱症，導火線則是與多年閨密陳珮騏鬧翻，她前不久接受媒體訪問，當聽見「陳珮騏」突然火大猛譙：「臭X，為了一個沒出息的男人和我撕破臉！」](#120)

At the upper level of the news text superstructural hierarchy, Example 11 topicalises the well-known Taiwan boy band in the subject position, and emotively points to "explosive allegations" about it. It contradictorily indicates that this is, at once, unpredictable ("surprising") and with precedence ("again"). Thereafter, it proximally links the lead singer's depression to the band's split and his sexual assault of a woman actor. In like manner, Example 12 topicalises the celebrity in the subject position, and emotively draws on the explosive trope ("fuse"/"fire"). It also indicates that the ill celebrity behaves unpredictably ("suddenly"). The paragraph proximally links the celebrity's depression to her long-standing disappearance, spiteful break-up with a close friend, and incongruous rage and abuse that would violate normative femininity in Chinese culture (Croll 1995; Guo 2010). Attention-grabbing, sensational reporting of this type only further casts those with a severe mental illness as volatile, erratic, unreliable, transgressive, and sexually suspect, in line with long-standing Chinese cultural stigma.

This apparent tension in the *Liberty Times* celebrity reports between more sensitive, magnanimous reporting on severe mental illness by way of inspirational testimony and more sensational and, so, commercially valuable, reporting of celebrity tattletale is also borne out by their atypical length. Across the entire corpus, *Liberty Times* reports, on average, are much shorter than their *People's Daily* and *Ming Pao* counterparts. Yet, most of its celebrity reports continue on at length from their reporting of the main event of the news story. They do so by further narrating the celebrities' troubled lives when ill; citing supportive comments from their colleagues, agents, fans, and family members; and listing details of their recent or upcoming appearances. The *People's Daily* celebrity reports also continue on at length from their reporting of the main event, as is typical of reports in this newspaper. At this lower level of the news text superstructural hierarchy, they present detailed life stories of celebrities with a severe mental illness or of other unrelated celebrities. At times, these life stories can be salacious. Interestingly, those that recount such details, without exception, report on women celebrities with a severe mental illness who reside outside of mainland China, namely, in Hong Kong, Taiwan, and Singapore. This locates any untoward reported behaviours and actions in geographical settings that have long been deemed by the mainland authorities to be morally corrupted by bourgeois liberal attitudes and thinking.

Most of the *Ming Pao* celebrity reports, by contrast, do not continue on from their reporting of the main event of the news story.

In sum, the *Ming Pao* and *Liberty Times* celebrity reports give greater voice to people with a severe mental illness. By contrast, their *People's Daily* counterparts do not. They, instead, maintain an orthodox biomedical air. The reports from all three newspapers, however, discursively deny celebrities with schizophrenia a voice. This likely is because schizophrenia is the most troubling of all mental illnesses in Chinese culture (Pearson 1996). Pearson (1996) states:

> Of all conditions, mental illness is one that confounds a culture that values conformity, discretion, modesty, and rectitude. The potential for disorder and nonconformity that severe mental disorder represents – particularly the symptoms of mania and schizophrenia – is deeply disturbing within Chinese society. Stigma and rejection of the mentally ill are common experiences in most societies, but in China they seem to be felt with a particular intensity.
>
> (p. 438)

Gender clearly shapes many of the *Ming Pao* and *Liberty Times* celebrity reports. Lurid, sensationally negative life stories are more likely to be about women celebrities with a severe mental illness. Conversely, inspirationally positive life stories, where celebrities overcome their illness, mostly depression, and return to society in a productive capacity, are exclusively about men. Women do not feature. What is more, these men successfully overcome their depression in ways that align with normative masculinity in Chinese culture.

This lopsided conjoining of women and negative outcomes in depression is reminiscent of the suicide reports that are analysed in Chapter 3. They, too, disproportionately link Chinese women to negative outcomes in depression, namely ignominious suicide. This occurs despite statistics that show that Chinese men with depression commit suicide more often than Chinese women with the illness across greater China. This lopsided focus on women with a severe mental illness adds further weight to the claim made in Chapter 3 (see section on suicide reports) that it may be less problematic to negatively report on women with a severe mental illness, due to the traditionally subordinate statuses of both women and severe mental illness in Chinese culture (Croll 1995; Louie 2002; Ramsay 2008, 2013, 2016; Shi-xu 2014).

The analysis of the celebrity reports has uncovered a tension between sensitive, magnanimous reporting on severe mental illness, in ways that humanise and empower those with the illness; and sensational, commercial-oriented reporting on the illness, in ways that bear out the long-standing stigmatic cultural construction of those with the illness as marginalised, unpredictable non-persons, who are best removed from everyday society. This tension is most evident in the *Liberty Times* reports. They are uncharacteristically long. This allows them to make full use of the attention-grabbing attraction of the celebrities. Moreover, a similar number of these reports recount sensationally negative circumstances in severe mental illness as recount inspirationally positive circumstances. This occurs across all levels of the news text superstructural hierarchy. As a result, the *Liberty Times* celebrity reports are just as likely to confirm the intense stigma against severe mental illness in Chinese culture as contest it. Such a tension also characterises the *Liberty Times* reports on crime and social wronging where severe mental illness is at issue, which are analysed in Chapter 3. Here, magnanimous topical, grammatical, and lexical sensitivities accompany luridly sensational reporting.

The *People's Daily* celebrity reports remain distinct from their *Ming Pao* and *Liberty Times* counterparts. They maintain a narrower focus on severe mental illness as a homogeneous biomedical concern, rather than a heterogeneous individual experience. This denies people with the illness agency. Doing so likely marks severe mental illness out as something that the state, alone, has the capability and the resources to readily address. The political agenda, therefore, is conspicuous in the *People's Daily* reports once again. This agenda also may explain why none of the celebrities with a severe mental illness who socially transgress in these reports, sometimes in very lurid ways, are from mainland China. This way, the reports maintain political correctness. The mainland authorities officially frown on the reporting of local celebrity tattletale (Shepherd 2017). Chapter 5 further examines how political forces and phenomena shape reporting on severe mental illness in the Chinese-language newspapers.

Reports on everyday personal experience

Everyday life stories provide useful insight into the illness experience for laypeople (see the earlier section on the voice of the lifeworld in this chapter). Despite this, all three Chinese-language newspapers appear to deprioritise reports that narrate the life stories of everyday people, as opposed to celebrities, who have a severe mental illness. Most starkly, there are no such reports in the *People's Daily* over its extended twelve-month period of analysis (see Appendix 1). It seems that the voice of everyday people with a severe mental illness in mainland China is most unwelcome in, or of little strategic use to, this newspaper. The *Ming Pao* and *Liberty Times* both have comparatively low proportions of reports on the everyday personal experience of the illness (see Appendices 2 and 3). The proportions are equal to or less than those for their celebrity reports, respectively.

The reports in both newspapers give near equal attention to people with a severe mental illness regardless of their gender. Most of them have depression (see Appendices 2 and 3). Moreover, most of them are young in the *Ming Pao* reports, while no age group dominates their *Liberty Times* counterparts. The *Ming Pao* suicide reports also disproportionately focus on young people with a severe mental illness. It is likely that young people having severe mental illness is more attention-grabbing than older people having the illness. The life stories of people with the illness are told by reporter-interviewers, health professionals, family caregivers, or friends, in descending frequency. First-hand accounts by those with the illness are uncommon.

The publication of the *Ming Pao* reports is quite evenly spread across each month, while that of their *Liberty Times* counterparts strongly cluster in March (see Appendices 2 and 3). There is no apparent reason for this cluster, with all of the March reports published before the brutal random killing of a young girl in Taipei late in this month (see section on crime reports in Chapter 3). The reports in both newspapers appear in a range of sections of the newspapers, namely, special columns, local news, lifestyle news, education news, and finance news, in descending frequency (see Appendices 2 and 3).

The headlines of the *Ming Pao* reports on the everyday personal experience of severe mental illness commonly name the illness at this highest level of the news text superstructural hierarchy (see selected Examples 13 and 14). This points to its newsworthiness.

13. Learn To "Humble Oneself" – Tang How-Kong Walks Away From Depression [學縮細「自我」 鄧厚江走出抑鬱] (#49)
14. Young Mother Suffered From Depression: Tried To Bang Head Against Wall [曾患抑鬱年輕媽媽：試過撼頭埋牆] (#83)

The headlines of their *Liberty Times* counterparts also do so, but only where the people, whose life stories are later recounted, have schizophrenia or generic severe mental illness, translated in Example 16 by way of the orthodox biomedical expression "psychiatric" (see selected Examples 15 and 16 below). Depression, seemingly, is less attention-grabbing than these two illnesses.

15. Helping Each Other In Illness – Schizophrenic Mother, Daughter Fight Serious Disease [疾病相扶持 思覺失調母女抗病魔] (#148)
16. Life In The Nursing Station – Psychiatric Ward [人生護理站 精神病房] (#185)

The headlines of the *Ming Pao* and *Liberty Times* reports also are gendered in different ways. The *Ming Pao* headlines regularly give positive agency to men with a severe mental illness, but not to women with the illness. In Example 13, the named man constructively, and admirably, "learns to humble himself" and "walks away from depression." By contrast, the unnamed woman with depression in Example 14 self-harms. She, tellingly, is designated by way of an esteemed familial role in normative Chinese femininity, namely, "mother." Mothers should not self-harm in normative Chinese femininity. The *Liberty*

Times headlines, on the other hand, regularly give positive agency to both women and men with a severe mental illness, although this is somewhat tempered when they have schizophrenia, an intensely stigmatised illness in Chinese culture. In Example 15, the women with schizophrenia – denoted by the neologism *sijueshitiao* – constructively, and admirably, "help each other" and "fight." This is reminiscent of the man with depression in the *Ming Pao* headline (Example 13). While fighting is traditionally a masculine pursuit in Chinese culture (Louie 2002; Lu 2012), the two women, contradictorily, are designated by way of esteemed familial roles in normative Chinese femininity, namely, "mother" and "daughter." The woman in the *Ming Pao* headline also is designated in this way (Example 14). Example 15, however, not only genders the two women in a narrow, culturally prescriptive way, but it also names them, in an essentialising way, through their illness. In like manner, Example 16 disempowers the woman with a severe mental illness, whose life story is later recounted, by locating her in a prison-like institution, removed from everyday society. This accords with stigmatic expectations in Chinese culture.

All of the *Ming Pao* reports on the everyday personal experience of severe mental illness, and all but two of their *Liberty Times* counterparts, lack discrete lead paragraphs. Instead, the opening paragraph of the news story in these reports either synopsises the life story of severe mental illness that is fully narrated in the lower levels of the news text superstructural hierarchy, or points to the reason for narrating this story (see selected Examples 17–19).

17. "If I hadn't come across a bass cello, I might have committed suicide due to the effects of depression." Twenty-six-year-old Charlie Wong lost his mother at a young age and had a bad relationship with his father. He turned to playing the cello as a release, but had no money to pay for tuition fees. Fortunately, his music teacher paid them for him. He studied and worked when at high school, toiling all night just to cover his living expenses. Once again, a kind teacher took on his tuition fees, and he successfully passed the Level 8 qualifying examination. After several twists and turns, he entered the Academy of Performing Arts, majoring in the bass cello and obtaining a scholarship. He will graduate in the coming year, and hopes to join a professional orchestra and be self-sufficient. This way, he can pay back the teachers who once offered him a helping hand. [「沒有遇上低音大提琴，我可能受抑鬱症影響到要輕生。」26 歲的王梓豪（Charlie）年幼喪母、與父親關係差、藉拉琴解愁但沒錢交學費，幸得音樂老師代為繳交；高中時半工讀，「返通宵更」掙生活費，又得良師「收平學費」，成功考得八級資格，幾經轉折入讀演藝學院主修低音大提琴，並獲獎學金。來年他即將畢業，希望投身專業樂團，自力更生，報答曾施以援手的老師。] (#42)

18. A woman from Taiwan by the name of Tseng and a man of Chinese nationality by the name of Lee got married. After spending half a year of happy times in Taiwan, they moved to mainland China to live. Ms Tseng suffered

from depression after having a miscarriage. In 2008, with great difficulty, she became pregnant with a daughter. Mr Lee actually tried to force her to have an abortion on the grounds of mainland China's one-child policy, but she refused. Since returning to Taiwan to give birth to her daughter, her husband has shown no interest in them. Ms Tseng relies on selling roasted sweet potatoes to support her darling daughter. The year before last, she filed for divorce with Shihlin District Court. A few days ago, the court ruled in her favour. [台灣曾姓女子和中國籍李姓男子結婚，在台灣度過半年甜蜜時光後，搬到中國定居，曾女因流產而罹憂鬱症，97年好不容易懷了女兒，李男竟以中國實施一胎化政策為由，逼她墮胎，曾女不從，回台生下女兒，丈夫從此不聞不問，曾女靠著賣烤地瓜養活寶貝女兒，前年向士林地院訴請離婚，法院日前判准。] (#152)

In Example 17 from *Ming Pao*, the man with depression, Charlie, gains voice at the outset of the paragraph, albeit fleeting. The synopsis of Charlie's upcoming life story is promptly taken over by the reporter-interviewer. Charlie's quote, nevertheless, foreshadows his positive agency in depression, most notably his mastering of a musical instrument. This remains the central topic of the entire paragraph. Men gaining positive agency despite their illness is typical of the reports on their everyday experience of severe mental illness, at this upper level of the news text superstructural hierarchy. Through conscientious, diligent effort, men are able to overcome the misery of severe mental illness to become productive members of everyday society. Charlie faces the torment of depression, suicidal thoughts, the death of his mother at a young age, family conflict, and abject poverty. Yet, through hard work, he is able to successfully support and educate himself, and master the bass cello. Moreover, he dutifully remembers and honours those who supported him in his life endeavour. This is what good men do in Chinese culture (Louie 2002; Lu 2012).

Example 18 from *Liberty Times* similarly topicalises the woman with depression, Ms Tseng, while a reporter-interviewer tells her story. The report consistently gives her positive agency that bears out her normative femininity in Chinese culture. Despite great hardship and obstacles, she admirably perseveres in getting pregnant and giving birth to a daughter, whom she treats in a motherly way as her little "darling." She also laudably provides for and rears the child on her own, without any support from her uncaring husband, whom she actively and successfully divorces. Giving positive agency to women and men with a severe mental illness is typical of the *Liberty Times* reports at this upper level of the news text superstructural hierarchy. Also typical is their displacing of blame for severe mental illness away from those with the illness, and onto antecedent factors and forces that appear to be beyond their control (Tolton 2009). The *Liberty Times* crime reports also do this. Ms Tseng develops depression after having a miscarriage. In other corresponding *Liberty Times* reports, both women and men develop severe mental illness after contracting cancer, working too hard, experiencing parental death at a young age, caring for a child with an intractable disease, and living with a parent who has a severe, long-standing gambling addiction.

By contrast, the *Ming Pao* reports on women's experiences of severe mental illness typically point to the personal failures of women, or the positive agency of others, at this upper level of the news text superstructural hierarchy (see selected Example 19).

19. In the summer of 2010, a group of clinical psychologists and reporter Vivian Tam started up the "Psychologist" column in *Sunday Ming Pao*. They wrote stories about people who are suffering from a severe mental illness or an emotional disorder. One of the interviewees, Ah Ching, had been troubled by an emotional disorder since high school, living between options of living or dying. She, nevertheless, created many "small worlds and friends" to help her overcome her negative moods. Ah Ching later emigrated. This Christmas, she has briefly returned to Hong Kong, and shares her unfinished story with readers. [2010年夏天，一班臨牀心理學家與記者譚蕙芸在《星期日生活》展開了「心理醫生」欄目，書寫受精神病/情緒病困擾的人的故事。當中一位受訪者阿晴，自高中開始受情緒病困擾，生活在生死選擇之間，然而她卻創造了 很多「小宇宙與朋友們」幫助自己克服負面情緒。阿晴後來移民，這個聖誕節， 她短暫回港，並跟讀者分享她未完的故事。] (#93)

This example puts discursive focus on the reporter-interviewer, Vivian Tam, and her colleagues from the mental health profession, from the outset of the paragraph. Making mention of the health experts adds credence and status to the newspaper column that is set up with their assistance. It also justifies the reporter telling Ah Ching's life story of severe mental illness on her behalf. Ah Ching, accordingly, is passively dubbed an "interviewee." She also lacks grammatical agency in "being troubled by an emotional disorder." This is typical of the *Ming Pao* reports on women's experiences of severe mental illness, at this upper level of the news text superstructural hierarchy. Women with the illness lack both voice and agency. This is not the case for men with the illness in the corresponding *Ming Pao* reports; and typically not so for both women and men with the illness in the corresponding *Liberty Times* reports. Also typical of the *Ming Pao* reports on women's experiences of severe mental illness at this upper level of the news text superstructural hierarchy is a consistent casting of their experience of severe mental illness in bleak and unsettled terms, with very few personal triumphs. Ah Ching's experience of her illness, which she later reveals is depression, is repeatedly marked by distress, indecision, death, negativity, flux, and incompleteness. By contrast, Charlie's and Ms Tseng's sad times in Examples 17 and 18 are more transitory, as they swiftly chalk up achievements and successes. This presages life stories that are linear in positive ascension. Ah Ching gains some agency later in Example 19, through "creating" support mechanisms, "emigrating," and "sharing" her life story. However, women like her, such as the young woman with depression in

Example 14 who self-harms, only gain positive agency at the lower levels of the news text superstructural hierarchy, in corresponding *Ming Pao* reports.

The discursive forms of the people's life stories of severe mental illness become clearer as they are narrated in the lower levels of the news text superstructural hierarchy. Across both the *Ming Pao* and the *Liberty Times* reports, a greater majority of these life stories give positive agency to people as they successfully overcome the challenge of their illness. Many of these stories also give voice to those with the illness, for the first time. This humanises them, albeit at a subordinate level of the news text superstructural hierarchy.

People with a severe mental illness achieve success in their life stories through diligence and hard work alone, in an apparent absence of biomedical intervention; or in the wake of intervention by health professionals. Success that follows diligence and hard work alone is typical for men with depression in the *Ming Pao* reports. This aligns with the narrative synopses in the upper levels of the news text superstructural hierarchy. Success that follows biomedical intervention is more common for women with depression, as well as women and men with schizophrenia (see selected Examples 20–22). This differs from the narrative synopses in the upper levels of the news text hierarchy, where success does not feature in the lives of women with depression and people with schizophrenia.

20. After the daughter was admitted to hospital she was definitively diagnosed with schizophrenia. After taking medication, her condition stabilised. Following treatment, she was referred to the youth mental health services at Stewards "Youth Outlook" in Hong Kong. After joining the group, Feng's daughter reconnected with the outside world. She now has thrown herself into social work. [女兒入院後確診思覺失調，服藥後情況穩定，經治療後轉介至香港神託會「青年新領域」青少年精神健康服務。馮的女兒參與小組後重新和外界接軌，現已投身社會工作。] (#75)
21. Every day I go in and out of the centre of Wan Chai and take part in various activities. I really want to be successful at this place. In the past six months, there have been two opportunities to return to the place at Prince Edward Road West, for volunteer work. I remember, back then, queuing to see the doctor at Kowloon Hospital. The things in Kowloon are delicious. I hope that I can return to that place in Kowloon every year and, along the way, eat to my heart's content. Although I have had a severe mental illness for ten years, I'm still in recovery [...] I hope that in the next ten years, I will be able to get along well with my friends and family. I also hope that I can be healthy and that everything goes well. [每天在灣仔的中心出入及參加各樣活動，很想在這個地方有一個成就。在剛過去的半年裏，有兩次機會因為義工的活動，回到太子道西這地方，又想起當年在九龍醫院排隊看病的情景。九龍的東西很好吃，我希望每年也順道回到九龍的地方吃個痛快。雖然有了十年精神病，自己仍在康復中。。。望在這未來的十年裏，能夠和朋友及親戚和睦相處，也望自己身體健康，事事如意。] (#43)

22. <u>Later on, I did the most detestable thing, so I continued to take my medication</u> [...] <u>Finally</u>, I chose to be <u>admitted to hospital</u>. If I didn't go, I might not have had the chance to see my son grow up. The child protection agency in Australia felt that I was unable to care for my baby. It wanted to take my son away. It said: "You are not qualified to be called a mother" [...] <u>In the end, [the hospital] report was good</u>. It said that <u>I dearly love my son, and the child protection agency slowly withdrew</u>. [後來我就做最憎的事，繼續吃藥。。。最後我選擇入院，如果我不去，我可能沒有機會看兒子成長。澳洲的保護兒童部門覺得我無法照顧BB，要帶走我的兒子，他說，「you are not qualified to be called a mother」。。。最後報告寫得很好，說我很疼兒子，保護兒童部門就慢慢退出。] (#93)

In Example 20, the life story of schizophrenia – denoted by the neologism *sijueshitiao* – lexically marks the temporal and, by implication, causal relationship ("after"/"following" > "now") between the young woman's contact with biomedical services and her successful return to society in a productive capacity. She demonstrates this in her life story by "reconnecting with the outside world" and "throwing herself into social work." Returning to society in a productive capacity can restore the personhood that those with a severe mental illness lose when acutely symptomatic (Guo 2016; Kleinman, Yan, Jun et al. 2011; Rosenberg 2018). This example further restricts attention to the young woman with schizophrenia and the biomedical institution that heals her. Regular use of passive voice and nominalisation grammatically conceals the identities of who admitted her to hospital, who diagnosed her, who gave her medication, who gave her treatment, and who referred her on to Stewards. This is typical of orthodox biomedical discourse (Candlin 2001; Dixon-Woods 2001; Fleischman 2003; Mishler 1984; Ramsay 2008; Samovar & Porter 2001. See introductory section of Chapter 1). It is biomedicine as a complex or institution that heals the young woman, not the actions of individual people. In doing so, biomedicine enables her to return to society in a productive capacity. With her personhood "now" restored, she gains grammatical agency ("joins"/"re-connects"/"throws herself into"). Despite granting her agency at this lower level of the news text superstructural hierarchy, the *Ming Pao* report continues to name her, in a disempowering and patriarchal way, as a grammatical possession of her father ("Feng's daughter").

In Example 21, the life story of schizophrenia – denoted earlier on in the report by the neologism *sijueshitiao* – links a young man's current success in recovery with a past biomedical intervention at Kowloon Hospital. His romanticises this intervention by coupling it to his memories of the locality's culinary delights. His diligent work ethic and noble future goals, seemingly, restore the personhood that he would have lost when symptomatic. As a result, he gains voice ("I") and grammatical agency ("go in and out"/"take part"/"get along"), at this lower level of the news text superstructural hierarchy. His, in my opinion, insightful first-hand account of life with schizophrenia, however, is preceded by, and followed by, a much longer account by his mother. This diminishes the import of his account in this *Ming Pao* report. His mother further points out, in a disempowering way, that she had made him write his account. She also devalues it and his self-of-now in recovery, by declaring, probably with the best of intentions, that his writing "still has large gaps in timing and logic, compared to before he got ill" [時序鋪排和邏輯思維方面，仍與以前病發前有很大的落差]. Moreover, she overlooks the valuable insight his first-hand account gives, narrowly calling attention to "the welcomed awareness that he now has of his illness and medication" [感恩的是他對自己的病和藥物有了認知]. In so doing, she gives precedence to the biomedical imperative over her own son's voice from the lifeworld.

The life story of depression recounted in Example 22, like that of schizophrenia recounted in Example 20, lexically marks the temporal and, by implication, causal relationship ("finally"/"in the end") between the woman's contact with biomedical services and her successful return to her normatively feminine role of mothering. The example, also like Example 20, orthodoxly casts biomedicine as a complex or institution, through its use of passive voice ("be admitted") and nominalisation ("the report"). Similar to Example 21, the woman, who recently emigrated from Hong Kong to Australia, gains grammatical agency ("take"/"chose"/"love") at this lower level of the news text superstructural hierarchy. Her reclaiming of her motherhood and, thus, her personhood, in this *Ming Pao* report, also restores her voice ("I") in an empowering way.

Women with depression and women and men with schizophrenia, therefore, gain agency and voice in the *Ming Pao* reports on the everyday personal experience of severe mental illness, but only at the lower levels of the news text superstructural hierarchy. Gaining agency is causally contingent upon biomedical intervention. Men with depression, by contrast, gain agency at higher levels of the news text superstructural hierarchy. Moreover, they do so without explicit mention of biomedical intervention. Acceding to biomedical intervention may be less problematic for the women in these reports since subordination to others is a key facet of normative femininity in Chinese culture (Croll 1995; Guo 2010). It also may be so for people with schizophrenia, given that they are stigmatically cast as non-persons in Chinese culture (Guo 2016; Kleinman, Yan, Jun et al. 2011; Wu 2010). By contrast, acceding to biomedical intervention may be more problematic for the men in these reports, since it does not tally with their masculine agency in overcoming adversity on their own. That is, unless they have schizophrenia.

The life stories of women and men with a severe mental illness in the *Liberty Times* reports, on the other hand, are more consistent across the upper and lower levels of the news text superstructural hierarchy. Across both of these levels, women and men with depression succeed in overcoming adversity through hard work, without explicit biomedical intervention. People with schizophrenia, however, never do. Gender, therefore, does not seem to shape the reporting of life stories of severe mental illness like it does in their *Ming Pao* counterparts. The *Liberty Times* reports, nevertheless, more frequently recount life stories where those with a severe mental illness live out their day-to-day lives in prison-like institutions, removed from everyday society (see selected Example 23 below). This is as Chinese cultural stigma would have it.

23. She yelled and screamed <u>in the hospital</u>, refusing to take her medication. The <u>nurse and orderly had no choice</u> but to <u>restrain</u> her. They pushed her into the <u>safe room</u>, and <u>tied up her hands and feet</u>. They only untied her when she had calmed down. Her <u>ward-mates</u> yelled and screamed, as they watched her <u>get locked up</u>. They were very sympathetic. After she was <u>released</u>, they huddled around her, urging her to: "Be good and take your medicine. You'll be okay!" [她在病院裡大喊大叫而且拒絕服藥，護佐與護士不得已只好將她架住，推進了保護室裡去，將她的手腳綁起來，等到她冷靜下來了，才給她鬆綁。病友們看著她被關時大喊大叫，都很同情，等她被釋放出來後，將她團團圍住勸告著：「妳乖乖吃藥就沒事了嘛！」] (#146)

Example 23 creates a prison-like hospital atmosphere, describing institutionally branded staff, namely "nurses and orderlies," who impersonally "restrain," "tie up," "lock up," and "release" those in their professional care, just as prison guards do. They also force those in their care, institutionally labelled as "ward-mates" (cf. cell-mates), into cell-like "safe rooms." This is because some ward-mates can be violent and uncooperative, as prison cell-mates often are. Accordingly, there are strict rules that hospital staff, like prison guards, "have no choice" but to enforce. If ward-mates abide by them, all "will be okay." All of them know the undisputed rationale behind these rules, namely, that pharmacotherapy heals.

In sum, all three Chinese-language newspapers appear to thematically deprioritise reporting on the everyday personal experience of severe mental illness. Just over one in ten reports in *Ming Pao* and *Liberty Times* recount life stories of everyday people with the illness, while no *People's Daily* reports do. By silencing lay voices, the *People's Daily* can maintain a greater focus on the authoritative state's preferred political agenda. Lay voices may implicitly or explicitly question this agenda.

The *Ming Pao* and *Liberty Times* reports on the everyday personal experience of severe mental illness construct the illness in ways that selectively

- uphold gender norms in Chinese culture.
- endorse the biomedical explanatory model of severe mental illness, in particular, that recovery from the illness is contingent on pharmacotherapeutic intervention and compliance.
- point to a hierarchy of illness, with schizophrenia the most marginalised illness.

- reveal a tension between sensitive, magnanimous reporting on severe mental illness, in ways that humanise and empower those with the illness; and sensational, commercial-oriented reporting on the illness, in ways that bear out the long-standing stigmatic cultural construction of those with the illness.

The *Ming Pao* reports gender the everyday experience of severe mental illness in ways that their *Liberty Times* counterparts do not. Men in the *Ming Pao* reports admirably and honourably overcome their illness in ways that align with normative masculinity in Chinese culture. This occurs at all levels of the news text superstructural hierarchy. Women with the illness, however, only do so at the lower levels of the news text superstructural hierarchy, and in ways that align with normative femininity in Chinese culture. The *Ming Pao* reports also gender pharmacotherapeutic intervention and compliance in severe mental illness. Men with depression seemingly succeed without pharmacotherapeutic intervention and compliance, while women with depression and women and men with schizophrenia only do so in the wake of such intervention and compliance. This not only selectively subordinates women but also people with schizophrenia, in ways that confirm cultural norms, values, and scripts.

The contingent linking of recovery from schizophrenia to pharmacotherapeutic intervention and compliance also characterises life stories about the illness that are published in a letters-to-the-editor-type section of a psychoeducational newsletter put out by a leading Beijing psychiatric hospital. My analysis of these life stories in Ramsay (2013) finds that they regularly contrast the disorder of a past life when acutely symptomatic with the relative order of a present life in recovery. This life in recovery is contingent on pharmacotherapeutic intervention and compliance. Doing so returns people with schizophrenia to their former selves. Now healed, they can return to society in a productive capacity. Successful pharmacotherapeutic intervention and compliance, in turn, require deferring to the authority of health professionals and embracing their biomedical explanatory model of severe mental illness at all times. An explanation that I pose in Ramsay (2013) for these discursive features of the psychoeducational life stories may also explain those of the *Ming Pao* reports on the everyday personal experience of severe mental illness. In Chinese culture, there is "a fundamental moral challenge" (Hydén 1995, p. 67) to provide for and protect those with schizophrenia; to ensure that they are not disruptive or threatening in public; and, where possible, to make them productive, functional citizens. Much of the burden for doing so still lies with the family members of those with schizophrenia (Pearson & Lam 2002; Ramsay 2013; Ran, Xiang, Simpson et al. 2005; Yang & Pearson 2002; Yip 2007). They need to dutifully defer to medical experts and people in authority, in line with prevailing Confucian-based norms, values, and scripts. By doing so, they can maintain a certain level of social face[1] amidst the culturally shameful circumstances that they find themselves in with schizophrenia. Accordingly, life stories of schizophrenia need to affirm a wholehearted familial commitment to a pharmacotherapeutic regimen that tames and subdues the socially feared person with schizophrenia. They also need to demonstrate esteem for and compliance with medical experts, who hold out the (questionable) promise of a future remedy that can allow those with schizophrenia to return to society in a productive capacity. The *Ming Pao* report that includes the voice of a mother, who is a family caregiver, and that of her son, who has schizophrenia, clearly demonstrates this discursive phenomenon. Her voice precedes his, in the upper level of the news text superstructural hierarchy. Here, she implicitly endorses pharmacotherapeutic intervention and compliance, in a face-gaining way. Her voice also reappears after her son's "lifeworld" voice (Mishler 1984, p. 104) (see earlier Example 21). Here, she implicitly diminishes and devalues what he says. As a result, attention remains on her and the healing biomedical explanatory model of severe mental illness.

Once again, the *Liberty Times* reports appear to humanise and empower those with a severe mental illness more than their *Ming Pao* counterparts do. Its reports are not normatively gendered, in disempowering ways. They also displace the blame for severe mental illness away from those with the illness and onto external factors and forces that appear to be beyond their control. This contests the long-standing stigmatic belief in Chinese culture that those with the illness are inherently tainted and, so, personally at fault. The *Liberty Times* reports, nevertheless, exhibit a tension between this more sensitive, magnanimous reporting, and that which is more sensational and commercial oriented. They relegate the voice of those with a severe mental illness to the lower levels of the news text superstructural hierarchy. As a result, they give greater weight to others' second-hand accounts of life in severe mental illness than to the first-hand accounts by those with the illness. The former typically endorse the biomedical explanatory model of severe mental illness (Ramsay 2013). The *Liberty Times* reports also document the lives of long-term patients in psychiatric hospitals more often than their *Ming Pao* counterparts do. Doing so validates long-standing stigmatic cultural attitudes and beliefs, which maintain that this is where people with a severe mental illness belong, removed from everyday society. Furthermore, the reports selectively make mention of schizophrenia, but not other forms of severe mental illness, at the highest level of the news text superstructural hierarchy, that is, the headline. This likely stems from the deemed sensational and, so, commercial value of doing so.

Life stories of severe mental illness

Reporting people's life stories can provide a more nuanced, diverse picture of severe mental illness, in opposition to the orthodox biomedical one that often dominates in today's world. More specific to the current study, it can usefully counterbalance the dominance of sensational reporting on crime and social wrongdoing where severe mental illness is at issue (*Ming Pao* and *Liberty Times*); or impersonal reporting on current medical findings about and government policy on the illness (*People's Daily*). This is because reporting people's life stories in severe mental illness can give them greater voice. Through their voice, a reader can more fully get to know the meanings that they ascribe to their illness. These meanings may emerge through their narration of time, causality, and identity, as well as the language that they use in their life stories (Ramsay 2013, 2016).

Many of the life stories of people with severe mental illness, be they well-known celebrities or everyday people, call attention to the moral and material successes of these people despite their illness. As such, the life stories function as inspirational testimonies. They have succeeded despite severe mental illness, so you can too. A key way that these life stories seek to positively inspire is by drawing attention to two distinct time periods in the lives of those with a severe mental illness, namely, life when acutely symptomatic, which is exceedingly dire, and life in recovery, where moral and material achievements abound. Accordingly, life when ill is "bad'" or "sad" (Whitley, Adeponle, & Miller 2015, p. 331), while life in recovery shows honour, courage, and diligence. The life stories also articulate conventionally gendered identities during these focal time periods. Men with depression inspirationally succeed in a normatively masculine way in the *Ming Pao* reports, at all levels of the news text superstructural hierarchy. This contrasts with Galasiński's (2008) discourse analysis of Polish men's life stories of depression, where the illness "undermines the dominant model of masculinity to the extent that a positive 'articulation' is impossible" (p. 133). Women with depression and women and men with schizophrenia in the *Ming Pao* reports, meanwhile, resolutely fail, or valiantly succeed but only in the lower levels of the news text superstructural hierarchy. Women and men with depression, on the other hand, inspirationally succeed in ways that align with gender norms in the *Liberty Times* reports, except when the women are celebrities. This occurs at all levels of the news text superstructural hierarchy. When women with a severe mental illness resolutely fail, they do so in ways that transgress normative femininity in Chinese culture.

This selective conjoining of women and failure in severe mental illness, which also characterises the suicide reports, may be traced to the subordinate statuses that women and the illness share in Chinese culture. As a result, it may be deemed less culturally confronting to recount a life story where a woman with a severe illness mental illness fails than one where a man with the illness fails. Conversely, an inspirational testimony about a man with a severe mental illness may carry greater import than one about a woman with the illness. By convention, social exemplars in Chinese culture are men (Jacka 2014; Roberts 2014).

While the *Ming Pao* reports more consistently gender in this way, they and their *Liberty Times* counterparts manifest a distinct binary, whereby those with a severe mental illness either valiantly succeed or fail dismally. Moreover, the reports from both newspapers consistently define success and failure through reductive cultural notions of social functioning and social worth. Those who succeed are culturally embodied and bestowed positive agency. As such, they counter the stigmatic cultural stereotype of people with a severe mental illness as unproductive, worthless non-persons (Guo 2016; Kleinman, Yan, Jun et al. 2011; Rosenberg 2018; Wu 2010). By contrast, those who fail are culturally disembodied and denied positive agency. They usually live apart from everyday society, as a marginal being or non-person. Such reporting aligns with readers' deep-seated beliefs about and attitudes towards them, that is, their "habits of mind" (Gibson & Jacobson 2018, p. 187).

This distinct binary is disempowering on two fronts. First, it maintains the stigmatic cultural stereotype, albeit only for some, but not all, people with a severe mental illness. Second, it maintains a "Chinese cultural prescription of social functioning, rather than individually-derived measures of achievement" (Ramsay 2013, p. 120. See also Kleinman, Yan, Jun et al. 2011; Ng, Pearson, Chen et al. 2011; Traphagan 2000). To demonstrate success, people with a severe mental illness need to "return to the community" [「回歸社區」], in a productive capacity. They have to do so at levels that, realistically, are beyond many of them, even when they are in recovery. Anything less than this, however, leaves them marked as culturally disembodied. Of course, by claiming that people with a severe mental illness are able to return to society in a productive capacity, the life stories counter their stigmatic cultural stereotype as unproductive, worthless non-persons. It is unfortunate, however, that these life stories must endorse a disempowering cultural prescription, namely, the productive Chinese citizen (Jacka 2014), in order to do so.

Whether people with a severe mental illness are successful or not, their life stories assign a cause for their illness. This differs somewhat across the three Chinese-language newspapers. The life stories in the *Ming Pao* reports, in a disempowering way, typically blame those with the illness. They are inherently flawed or tainted, in line with the stigmatic cultural stereotype. The life stories in the *Liberty Times* reports, by contrast, commonly direct blame away from those with the illness, and onto antecedent factors and forces that they appear to have no control over, some of which are social in origin. This contests the stigmatic cultural stereotype. The life stories in the *People's Daily* reports, meanwhile, more narrowly draw on an orthodox biomedical aetiological model in order to explain severe mental illness. In doing so, they regularly use biomedical lexis and reasoning. They also more commonly use the generic label for severe mental illness rather than specific diagnostic labels. The *People's Daily* crime reports also do this. Labelling severe mental illness in this way casts it as a homogeneous entity, "consolidat[ing] [...] the difference between normality and abnormality" (Georgaca & Bilić 2007, p. 175). The state and its affiliates are well prepared and well equipped to effectively meet the challenge that such an entity presents. As a result, the biomedical agenda and political agenda coalesce in these reports. Chapter 5 examines this discursive phenomenon in greater detail.

By narrating the life stories of severe mental illness in the ways outlined above, the reports in all three newspapers fail to give those with the illness a clear voice, unless they are a celebrity. Even then, others largely narrate their life stories, as uniformly is the case for everyday people with the illness. Their first-hand voice, seemingly, is suspect or of little value. When what those with a severe mental illness say is reported, it is relegated to the lower levels of the news text superstructural hierarchy. This is consistently and notably so in schizophrenia, the most "disturbing" of all mental illnesses in Chinese culture (Pearson 1996, p. 438). As a result, the life stories recounted in these reports drift away from Mishler's (1984, p. 104) emblematic "voice of the lifeworld." Instead, they more purposively satisfy commercial needs, while maintaining cultural and political status quos. This significantly diminishes their capacity to humanise, empower, and liberate a highly marginalised group of people across greater China.

Note

1 Face is a social phenomenon grounded in concern for "how one is evaluated by others" (Hinze 2002, p. 269). See also Shi-xu (2014).

References

Ainsworth-Vaughn, N. (2003). The discourse of medical encounters. In D. Schiffrin, D. Tannen, & H. E. Hamilton (Eds.), *The handbook of discourse analysis* (pp. 453–469). Oxford: Blackwell.

Angermeyer, M. C., & Schulze, B. (2001). Reinforcing stereotypes: How the focus on forensic cases in news reporting may influence public attitudes towards the mentally ill. *International Journal of Law and Psychiatry, 24*(4), 469–486.

Bhui, K., & Bhugra, D. (2002). Explanatory models for mental distress: Implications for clinical practice and research. *British Journal of Psychiatry, 181*, 6–7.

Blood, R. W., Putnis, P., & Pirkis, J. (2002). Mental-illness news as violence: A news frame analysis of the reporting and portrayal of mental health and illness in Australian media. *Australian Journal of Communication, 29*(2), 59–82.

Brady, A. (2008). *Marketing dictatorship: Propaganda and thought work in contemporary China*. Lanham, MD: Rowman & Littlefield.

Candlin, C. N. (2001). Medical discourse as professional and institutional action: Challenges to teaching and researching languages for special purposes. In M. Bax & C. J. Zwart (Eds.), *Reflections on language and language learning: In honour of Arthur Van Essen* (pp. 185–207). Amsterdam: John Benjamins.

Cashman, E. L., & Thomas. S. D. M. (2017). Does mental illness impact the incidence of crime and victimisation among young people? *Psychiatry, Psychology and Law, 24*(1), 33–46.

Chou, J. Y. (2006). *The psychiatric politics of risk and cost: Forensic theory and practice in the US and Taiwan* [Doctoral dissertation. Seattle, WA: University of Washington].

Clement, S., & Foster, N. (2008). Newspaper reporting on schizophrenia: A content analysis of five national newspapers at two time points. *Schizophrenia Research, 98*(1), 178–183.

Croll, E. (1995). *Changing identities of Chinese women: Rhetoric, experience and self perception in twentieth century China.* Hong Kong: Hong Kong University Press.

Dixon-Woods, M. (2001). Writing wrongs? An analysis of published discourses about the use of patient information leaflets. *Social Science and Medicine, 52*(9), 1417–1432.

Fleischman, S. (2003). Language and medicine. In D. Schiffrin, D. Tannen, & H. E. Hamilton (Eds.), *The handbook of discourse analysis* (pp. 470–502). Oxford: Blackwell.

Galasiński, D. (2008). *Men's discourses of depression.* London: Palgrave Macmillan.

Galasiński, D. (2013). *Fathers, fatherhood and mental illness: A discourse analysis of rejection.* London: Palgrave Macmillan.

Galasiński, D. (2017). *Discourses of men's suicide notes: A qualitative analysis.* New York: Bloomsbury Academic.

Garden, R. (2010). Telling stories about illness and disability: The limits and lessons of narrative. *Perspectives in Biology and Medicine, 53*(1), 121–135.

Georgaca, E., & Bilić, B. (2007). Representations of "mental illness" in Serbian newspapers: A critical discourse analysis. *Qualitative Research in Psychology, 4*(1), 167–186.

Gibson, C., & Jacobson, T. (2018). Habits of mind in an uncertain information world. *Reference and User Services Quarterly, 57*(3), 183–192.

Guo, J. (2016). *Stigma: An ethnography of mental illness and HIV/AIDS in China.* Hackensack, NJ: World Century.

Guo, Y. (2010). China's celebrity mothers: Female virtues, patriotism and social harmony. In L. Edwards & E. Jeffreys (Eds.), *Celebrity in China* (pp. 45–66). Hong Kong: Hong Kong University Press.

Harper. D. J. (1995). Discourse analysis and 'mental health'. *Journal of Mental Health, 4*, 347–357.

Harper. D. J. (1996). Deconstructing 'Paranoia': Towards a discursive understanding of apparently unwarranted suspicion. *Theory and Psychology, 6*(3), 423–448.

Hinze, C. (2002). *Re-thinking 'face': Pursuing an emic-etic understanding of Chinese mian and lian and English face.* [Doctoral dissertation, University of Queensland].

Hsu, C. C., Sheu, C. J., Liu, S. I., Sun, Y. W., Wu, S. I., & Lin, Y. (2009). Crime victimization of persons with severe mental illness in Taiwan. *Australasian Psychiatry, 43*(5), 460–466.

Hunt, L. M. (2000). Strategic suffering: Illness narratives as social empowerment among Mexican cancer patients. In C. Mattingly & L. C. Garro (Eds.), *Narrative and the cultural construction of illness and healing* (pp. 88–107). Berkeley, CA: University of California Press.

Hurwitz, B. (2004). The temporal construction of medical narratives. In B. Hurwitz, T. Greenhalgh, & V. Skultans (Eds.), *Narrative research in health and illness* (pp. 414–427). Malden, MA: BMJ Books.

Hydén, L. C. (1995). In search of an ending: Narrative reconstruction as a moral quest. *Journal of Narrative and Life History, 5*(1), 67–84.

Hydén, L. C. (1997). Illness and narrative. *Sociology of Health and Illness, 19*(1), 48–69.

Hydén, L. C., & Brockmeier, J. (2008). Introduction: From the retold to the performed story. In L. C. Hydén & J. Brockmeier (Eds.), *Health, illness and culture: Broken narratives* (pp. 1–15). New York: Routledge.

Hydén, L. C., & Örulv, L. (2009). Narrative and identity in Alzheimer's disease: A case study. *Journal of Aging Studies, 23*(4), 205–214.

Jacka, T. (2014). Left-behind and vulnerable? Conceptualising development and older women's agency in rural China. *Asian Studies Review, 38*(2), 186–204.

Kleinman, A. (1988). *The illness narratives: Suffering, healing, and the human condition.* New York: Basic Books.

Kleinman, A., Yan, Y., Jun, J., Lee, S., Zhang, E., Pan, T., Wu, F., & Guo, J. (2011). *Deep China: The moral life of the person: What anthropology and psychiatry tell us about China today.* Berkeley, CA: University of California Press.

Lafrance, M. (2007). A bitter pill: A discursive analysis of women's medicalized accounts of depression. *Journal of Health Psychology, 12*(1), 127–140.

Louie, K. (2002). *Theorising Chinese masculinity: Society and gender in China.* Cambridge, UK: Cambridge University Press.

Louie, K. (2015). *Chinese masculinities in a globalizing world.* New York: Routledge.

Lu, Y. (2012). *Heroic masculinity and male homosociality in* Three Kingdoms *and* Le Morte Darthur [Doctoral dissertation, The University of Queensland].

Lung, F. W., Liao, S. C., Wu, C. Y., & Lee, M. B. (2017). The effectiveness of suicide prevention programmes: Urban and gender disparity in age-specific suicide rates in a Taiwanese population. *Public Health, 147*(2017), 136–143.

Lupton, D. (2003). *Medicine as culture: Illness, disease and the body in Western societies.* Thousand Oaks, CA: SAGE.

MacDonald, T. H. (1998). *Rethinking health promotion: A global approach.* London, New York: Routledge.

Mishler, E. G. (1984). *The discourse of medicine: Dialectics of medical interviews.* Norwood: Ablex.

Ng, R. M. K., Pearson, V., Chen, E. E. Y., & Law, C. W. (2011). What does recovery from schizophrenia mean? Perceptions of medical students and trainee psychiatrists. *International Journal of Social Psychiatry, 57*(3), 248–262.

Pearson, V. (1996). The Chinese equation in mental health policy and practice. *International Journal of Law and Psychiatry, 19*(3/4), 437–458.

Pearson, V., & Lam, P. (2002). On their own: Caregivers in Guangzhou, China. In H. Lefley & D. Johnson (Eds.), *Family interventions in mental illness: International perspectives* (pp. 171–183). Westport, CT: Praeger.

Ramsay, G. (2008). *Shaping minds: A discourse analysis of Chinese-language community mental health literature.* Amsterdam: John Benjamins.

Ramsay, G. (2010). Mainland Chinese family caregiver narratives in mental illness: Disruption and continuity. *Asian Studies Review, 34*(1), 83–103.

Ramsay, G. (2013). *Mental illness, dementia and family in China.* London: Routledge.

Ramsay, G. (2016). *Chinese stories of drug addiction: Beyond the opium dens.* New York: Routledge.

Ran, M. S., Xiang, M. Z., Simpson, P., & Chan, C. L. W. (2005). *Family-based mental health care in rural China.* Hong Kong: Hong Kong University Press.

Riessman, C. K. (2004). A thrice-told tale: New readings of an old story. In B. Hurwitz, T. Greenhalgh & V. Skultans (Eds.), *Narrative research in health and illness* (pp. 309–324). Malden, MA: BMJ Books.

Roberts, C., & Sarangi, S. (1999). Hybridity in gatekeeping discourse: Issues of practical relevance for the researcher. In S. Sarangi & C. Roberts (Eds.), *Talk, work and institutional order: Discourse in medical, mediation and management settings* (pp. 473–504). New York: Mouton de Gruyter.

Roberts, R. (2014). The Confucian moral foundation of socialist model man. *New Zealand Journal of Asian Studies, 16*(1), 23–38.

Rosenberg, A. (2018, 18 June). Hiding my mental illness from my Asian family almost killed me: The silent shame of having a mental illness in a Chinese family. *Vox.* www.vox.com/first-person/2018/6/18/17464574/asian-chinese-community-mental-health-illness.

Rukavina, T. V., Nawka, A., Brborović, O., Jovanović, N., Kuzman, M. R., Nawková, L., Bednárová, B., Zŭchová, S., Hrodková, M., & Lattova, Z. (2012). Development of the PICMIN (picture of mental illness in newspapers): Instrument to assess mental illness stigma in print media. *Social Psychiatry and Psychiatric Epidemiology, 47*(7), 1131–1144.

Samovar, L. A., & Porter, R. E. (2001). *Communication between cultures.* Belmont, CA: Wadsworth/Thomson Learning.

Sarangi, S. (1998). Institutional language. In J. L. Mey (Ed.), *Concise encyclopaedia of pragmatics* (pp. 382–385). Oxford: Elsevier.

Shepherd, C. (2017, 8 June). China closes 60 celebrity gossip social media accounts. *Reuters.* www.reuters.com/article/us-china-internet-censorship-idUSKBN18Z0J3

Shi-xu. (2014). *Chinese discourse studies.* Hampshire, UK: Palgrave Macmillan.

Sontag, S. (1989). *Illness as metaphor and AIDS and its metaphors.* New York: Picador.

Tang, L., & Bie, B. (2015). Narratives about mental illnesses in China: The voices of Generation Y. *Health Communication, 31*(2), 171–181.

Tolton, L. (2009). *Legitimation of violence against women in Colombia: A feminist critical discourse analytic study* [Doctoral dissertation. St Lucia, QLD: The University of Queensland].

Traphagan. J. W. (2000). *Taming oblivion: Aging bodies and the fear of senility in Japan.* New York: State University of New York Press.

Whitley, R., Adeponle, A., & Miller, A. R. (2015). Comparing gendered and generic representations of mental illness in Canadian newspapers: An exploration of the chivalry hypothesis. *Social Psychiatry and Psychiatric Epidemiology, 50* (2), 325–333.

Wu, F. (2010). *Suicide and justice: A Chinese perspective.* New York: Routledge.

Wu, H. Y. J., & Cheng, A. T. A. (2017). A history of mental healthcare in Taiwan. In H. Minas, & M. Lewis (Eds.), *Mental health in Asia and the Pacific: Historical and cultural perspectives* (pp. 107–121). Boston, MA: Springer.

Yang, L. H., & Pearson, V. J. (2002). Understanding families in their own context: Schizophrenia and structural family therapy in Beijing. *Journal of Family Therapy, 24*, 233–257.

Yip, K. S. (2007). *Mental health service in the People's Republic of China: Current status and future developments.* New York: Nova Science Publishers.

5 The establishment and severe mental illness

Chapters 3 and 4 find that *Ming Pao* and *Liberty Times* regularly appear to report on severe mental illness for sensational effect, the former more conspicuously so. This occurs even when these newspapers narrate life stories of those with a severe mental illness. As a result, the newspapers appear to forgo an opportunity to discursively empower, humanise, and liberate those with the illness by giving them a clear voice. Reporting in this way maintains the cultural and political status quos that characterise the geographical location where the newspaper is published. This chapter further examines the extent to which, how, and why reporting on severe mental illness in the three Chinese-language newspapers bears out and upholds key narratives that are championed by orthodox biomedical and political establishments. These elite narratives espouse preferred understandings of, and explanations for, severe mental illness, as well as wider issues of concern, such as the doctor-patient hierarchy, pharmacotherapeutic supremacy, social progress, social harmony, social stability, and the rule of law. The chapter considers the impact and import of these narratives, and their potential strategic use for political purpose. In doing so, it points out the extent to which, how, and why their use confirms or contests the intense prevailing stigma against severe mental illness in culturally Chinese communities.

Psychiatric amenities in present-day greater China

Across the globe, many practitioners of contemporary psychiatry embrace an orthodox doctor-centred biomedical approach to severe mental illness, as opposed to one that is more client-centred and mutually reflective. The introductory section of Chapter 1 and Chapter 4 section on the voice of the lifeworld define such an approach to the practice of clinical medicine, including psychiatry. Greater China is no exception. At present, mainland China has 728 dedicated psychiatric hospitals (Patel, Xiao, Chen et al. 2016; World Health Organization 2014). The number of dedicated psychiatric residential facilities is unknown, but anecdotally said to be few in number (World Health Organization 2014). On a per capita basis, the number of dedicated hospitals is twice that for Hong Kong, yet much lower than that for Taiwan. This points to mainland China's more traditional amalgam of an institution-centred approach to and management of severe mental illness (Xu, Li, Xu et al. 2017), alongside an ongoing constituted reliance on family care and supervision in the local community, relative to Hong Kong and Taiwan (Every-Palmer, Brink, Chern et al. 2014; Li, Gutheil & Hu 2016; Phillips, Chen, Diesfeld et al. 2013; Topiwala, Wang, & Fazel 2012; Xue, Shi, Knoll et al. 2015). As noted in the Chapter 2 section on the approaches to and management of severe mental illness in greater China over the ages, mainland China has a very low number of practicing psychiatrists per capita.

Hong Kong has just two dedicated psychiatric hospitals and forty-five dedicated psychiatric residential facilities (World Health Organization 2011). While, on a per capita basis, the number of psychiatric hospitals is lower than that for mainland China, Hong Kong retains an extensive, more highly developed network of local community mental health units. These units are located right across the special administrative region. This points to Hong Kong's more progressive client-centred approach to severe mental illness. Hong Kong has many more practicing psychiatrists than mainland China on a per capita basis, yet lags behind Taiwan and Western countries such as Australia (see section on the approaches to and management of severe mental illness in greater China over the ages in Chapter 2).

Taiwan has forty-four dedicated psychiatric hospitals and 141 dedicated psychiatric residential facilities (Ministry of Health & Welfare 2017). The number of dedicated hospitals per capita is far greater than that for mainland China and Hong Kong, while the number of dedicated residential facilities per capita corresponds to that for Hong Kong. This points to Taiwan's more orthodox, institution-centred approaches to and management of severe mental illness, relative to those adopted in mainland China and Hong Kong. As noted in the Chapter 2 section on the approaches to and management of severe mental illness in greater China over the ages, the number of practicing psychiatrists in Taiwan per capita equals that in Western countries such as Australia.

There is an inverse relationship between the level of development of psychiatric amenities in a geographical community and the frequency with which its resident Chinese-language newspaper reports on current medical findings about severe mental illness and related disorders, such as prevalence rates, causes, early warning signs, and treatments, as well as available support services and public health measures. Medical reports numerically rank first in the *People's Daily*. This is so for the six-month period that is common to all three newspapers, as well as the six-month period that precedes it. By contrast, medical reports numerically rank only sixth and third in *Ming Pao* and *Liberty Times*, respectively. These two newspapers give much greater thematic attention to crime where severe mental illness is implicated, and to the celebrity experience of the illness. This is especially so for *Ming Pao*. The ensuing discourse analysis clarifies and rationalises this apparent paradox, whereby the resident newspaper of the geographical community whose psychiatric amenities are least developed reports proportionally most frequently on psychiatric issues and related medical concerns.

Medical reports

Publication of the *People's Daily* and *Liberty Times* reports on current medical findings about severe mental illness and related disorders, such as prevalence rates, causes, early warning signs, and treatments, as well as available support services and public health measures, does not notably cluster in any one month (see Appendices 1 and 3). The medical reports in these two newspapers mostly deal with depression (see Appendices 1 and 3). They typically appear in specialist medical news or science news sections of these two newspapers (see Appendices 1 and 3). As a consequence, the *People's Daily* and *Liberty Times* schematically call attention to the elite status of biomedicine, by setting their medical reports apart from the seemingly ordinary news that is reported in their local news or national news sections. Their medical reports also more narrowly focus on a specific diagnosis, namely depression, as biomedicine would have it. Publication of the *Ming Pao* medical reports, by contrast, clusters in March and May of 2016 (see Appendix 2). There is no common factor that can explain these clusters. In addition, the medical reports appear in the newspaper's local news section or in special columns, rather than in specialist medical news or science news sections (see Appendix 2). They also more often report on generic severe mental illness than on depression (see Appendix 2). Georgaca and Bilić (2007) state that doing so more readily marginalises those with the illness, as an abnormal social group.

Like all social phenomena and experience, contemporary psychiatry is shaped by and informs a matrix of competing discourses. The orthodox doctor-centred voice of biomedicine, as opposed to one that is more client-centred and mutually reflective, typically colonises the headlines of the medical reports in all three Chinese-language newspapers. This voice upholds the biomedical explanatory model of severe mental illness "as a known or given reality," such that "the exact biochemical mechanism need not be explained" (Rowe, Tilbury, Rapley et al. 2003, p. 686). Doing so "reinforces the expert's position as expert, and the reader as either not needing proper explanation because of the expert's expertness, or because of their own inability to understand the technicalities of the biochemical processes" (Rowe, Tilbury, Rapley et al. 2003, p. 686). As a result, severe mental illness is "simultaneously" cast as "an underdetermined and overdetermined concept, being ill-defined and contentious, but also taken for granted as […] in need of cure through biological, psychological or social-structural means" (Rowe, Tilbury, Rapley et al. 2003, p. 693).

Accordingly, the headlines of the medical reports in all three Chinese-language newspapers regularly name people, in impersonal ways, through their illness, or the use of the reductive medical label "sufferer" (see selected Examples 1, 2, 4, and 5). They also typically use medical terminology and cause-and-effect coherence relations (see selected Examples 1, 2, and 5). Doing so harks back to the orthodox clinical narrative of symptoms > diagnosis > treatment. The headlines of the medical reports in all three newspapers further maintain the institutional tone of the orthodox voice of biomedicine. This results from their regular use of command modals and imperative clauses; prioritisation of the voice of authority; and the citing of statistics and the findings of scientific research (see selected Examples 1–6).

1 Schizophrenia Is Prone To Relapse – Needs Early, Ample, Specified Treatment [精神分裂症容易复发 需早期、足疗程规范治疗] (#6)
2 Our Nation's Severe Mental Illness Sufferers Reach 4.3 Million [我国严重精神病患者达430万人] (#16)
3 Watch Out If Feeling Down For 2 Weeks! [Down足兩星期，小心！] (#38)
4 Things You Should Know: Strictly Remember "3 No's" To Avoid Upsetting Sufferer [知多啲：緊記「三不」免刺激患者] (#66)
5 Taking Care Of Dementia Sufferers, Watch Out For Depression [照顧失智者 小心憂鬱症] (#103)
6 Research Finds Women More Easily Depressed Than Men [研究發現女比男更易憂鬱] (#113)

Examples 1 and 2 from the *People's Daily* additionally cast severe mental illness as a pressing medical concern for the mainland Chinese state and its affiliates, as a number of its other headlines do. By contrast, the headlines in the *Ming Pao* counterparts (Examples 3 and 4) and *Liberty Times* counterparts (Examples 5 and 6) do not. Instead, they cast severe mental illness as an apparent threat that everyday people need to be aware of and keep a sharp lookout for. Fortunately, strict pharmacotherapeutic compliance can prevent those with the illness from becoming overly disruptive, as they ordinarily are in long-standing Chinese stigmatic thinking (see selected Example 7).

7 Receive Treatment, Take Medication On Time – Schizophrenia Sufferers Won't Cause Trouble [接受治療 定期服藥 思覺失調患者不使壞] (#125)

None of the medical reports in all three Chinese-language newspapers have a summary lead paragraph. Their reporting of the main event of a news story consistently prioritises the agency of people in authority, such as government officials, university academics, medical researchers, and health professionals, over people with a severe mental illness. In doing so, they exhibit the orthodox biomedical-cum-institutional discursive features that characterise their headlines. Many reports start by recounting anecdotes about severe mental illness or posing questions about it, which people in authority subsequently comment on or answer. People with the illness never do. Instead, those in authority paternalistically "register" [登记在册], "control" [控制], "manage" [管理], "monitor" [監察], "experiment on" [做實驗], "intervene in" [干预], "guide" [疏导], "help" [助], and "rescue" [救] them. Those in authority also reductively name them as "sufferers/ patients" [病人], "cases" [個案], "groups" [組別/ 群体], "visits" [人次], "the deceased" [死者], and "a community of the mentally disordered" [精神障碍社区]. This diminishes their personhood, and makes it easier to marginalise them as a homogeneous social other. In like manner, those in authority clinically assemble the bodies of those with the illness by way of an orthodox biomedical lexicon, such as "symptom" [徵狀], "cognitive function" [認知功能], "definitive diagnosis" [確診], and object of "treatment" [治療]. They also logically cohere their lives using cause-and-effect markers, such as "as a result" [因而/ 結果], "lead to" [導致], "caused by" [所致], "because of" [因], "due to" [由于], and "cause" [令/ 让/ 造成/ 引起]. Such language and rhetoric typify the orthodox voice of biomedicine (Ramsay 2008). The medical reports in all three newspapers regularly nominalise dealings between those in authority and those with the illness. Doing so discursively erases the latter at this upper level of the news text superstructural hierarchy (Sarangi 1998) (see selected Examples 8–10).

8   <u>Experts</u> point out that the <u>onset</u> of schizophrenia is slow. It gradually progresses and the <u>course</u> of the disease is prolonged, with easy <u>relapse</u>. The complete <u>management</u> of the <u>course</u> of the disease should not only focus on <u>control</u> of the patient's symptoms during the acute phase. It also requires <u>paying attention to</u> the <u>fluctuations</u> in the patient's condition during the <u>consolidation</u> and <u>recovery</u> phases, and rendering appropriate <u>intervention</u> and <u>guidance</u> as early as possible. [专家指出，精神分裂症起病多缓慢，逐渐进展，病程迁延且容易复发，其全病程管理不仅要着眼于患者在急性期症状控制，更要关注巩固期和恢复期的患者病情的波动情况，尽早给予恰当的干预和疏导。] (#6)

9   The <u>Education Bureau</u> stated that it will maintain contact with the <u>Hospital Authority</u> to jointly examine and discuss strengthening the current <u>notification, referral,</u> and <u>support</u> mechanisms, and ensure cross-disciplinary <u>cooperation</u> and <u>communication</u>. [教育局表示與醫管局保持聯繫，共同檢視和商討加強現有通報、轉介和支援機制，確保跨專業的協作和溝通。] (#37)

10   Depression has been classified by the <u>World Health Organization</u> as the second most common disease to cause <u>incapacity</u> and premature <u>death</u> in the twenty-first century, being second only to cardiovascular disease. [憂鬱症已被世界衛生組織列為廿一世紀引起失能及早逝的第二位疾病，僅次於心血管疾病。] (#119)

Nominalisation of verbs in Example 8 from the *People's Daily*, Example 9 from *Ming Pao*, and Example 10 from *Liberty Times* discursively erases people with a severe mental illness, maintaining attention on those in authority, namely, the "experts," the Education Bureau, Hospital Authority, and World Health Organization, along with the illness labels that they favour. Example 8, alone, makes any mention of people with a severe mental illness. When it does, it names them using the reductive biomedical label "patient."

The label, furthermore, has a subordinate status in grammatically modifying the focal, illness-related nouns "symptoms" and "condition." Other *People's Daily* medical reports additionally call attention to the national (patriotic) duty of people with a severe mental illness to wholly submit to biomedical authorities and comply with pharmacotherapy, at this upper level of the news text superstructural hierarchy. By doing so, they can "return to the real world" [回归真实世界] from their seemingly unreal world of severe mental illness.

Most of the medical reports in *Ming Pao* and *Liberty Times* continue on to elaborate on the severe mental illness at issue. By contrast, only a small number of their *People's Daily* counterparts do. At this lower level of the news text superstructural hierarchy, the reporting in all three newspapers remains heavily colonised by the impersonal, reductive voices of biomedicine and institutional authority. The *People's Daily* medical reports additionally continue to call attention to the focal role of the state in severe mental illness. At this lower level of the news text superstructural hierarchy, they cast the illness as a "threat" [威胁] to the "nation" [我国/ 中国]. They do so by calling attention to the inherent "instability" [不稳定] of "sufferers" [患者] due to their "unsound or flawed temperaments" [性格不健全或有缺陷]. This makes them exhibit "dangerous behaviour that causes harm to themselves or others" [自残或者伤害他人的危险行为], as well as random "disturbances and accidents" [有肇事肇祸行为]. This has "bad effects on those around them, their surroundings, and their families" [对周围的人和环境家庭有一些不好的影响]. As a result, they remain "isolated from the outside world" [与外界环境隔绝], and "unable to live normally" [不能正常生活]. The state, thus, rightfully controls them, through structured "treatment in hospital" [治疗在医院], and "management in the community" [管理在社区]. This is especially important for those with schizophrenia, who have a proclivity to "reduce or stop taking medication on their own accord" [自行减药或停止用药]. The *Ming Pao* and *Liberty Times* medical reports similarly cast severe mental illness as a threat, but at higher levels of their news text superstructural hierarchy.

In sum, the medical reports in the three Chinese-language newspapers consistently prioritise the orthodox voice of biomedicine and the voice of institutional authority over that of people with a severe mental illness. This aligns with Chinese cultural norms and scripts, whereby laypeople accede to the advice and direction of those in authority with specialist knowledge (Ng 2000; Ramsay 2008, 2013; Shi-xu 2014; Zhuang, Wong, Cheng et al. 2017). A characteristically impersonal and reductive language and rhetoric objectify and disempower those with a severe mental illness, at all levels of the news text superstructural hierarchy. This bears out their cultural status as non-persons that are acted upon by others (Guo 2016; Kleinman, Yan, Jun et al. 2011; Rosenberg 2018; Wu 2010). Their voices remain silent, diminishing their agency as others count, monitor, examine, and experiment on their bodies.

The medical reports in all three newspapers, however, more variably cast people with a severe mental illness as a threat to the local community. Threats warrant urgent and diligent action. Accordingly, casting those with a severe mental illness as a threat legitimises their biomedical control and removal from everyday society. The *Ming Pao* and *Liberty Times* medical reports regularly do so, and at the upper levels of their news text superstructural hierarchy. Medical reports, nonetheless, only account for a low proportion of reports on severe mental illness in these two newspapers. By contrast, they account for the highest proportion of reports in the *People's Daily*. Its reports less commonly cast people with a severe mental illness as a threat to the local community. Moreover, when they do so, it is at the lower levels of their news text superstructural hierarchy. This diminishes the impact of doing so. Instead, the *People's Daily* medical reports typically cast those with the illness as an undesirable, rather than an overtly feared, social group. The mainland Chinese state strategically and systematically uses biomedicine, policy, and the law to control, regulate, and correct this marginalised group of people, with the intention of returning them to society in a productive capacity. This greatly benefits them and the nation (Shi-xu 2014). Reporting in this way necessarily blurs the boundary between the practice of biomedicine and the operation of state policy and the law on the mainland.

By historical comparison, what drives this orthodox biomedicalisation of severe mental illness in the three Chinese-language newspapers differs from what drove its biomedicalisation in newspapers of the early Republican era. Baum (2018) states that the biomedical explanation was novel to Republican-era China. She points out that it was not the *reporting* in the Republican-era newspapers that "functioned as an initial means by which psychiatric and neurological discourses penetrated Chinese society," but their numerous "[a]dvertisements for anti-neurasthenic products and services" (2018, p. 103). Thus, simple commerce, rather than altruism or efforts to validate authoritative knowledge and power, "served to generate new forms of psychiatric knowledge" at the time (Baum 2018, p. 98). Baum (2018, p. 98) adds that this led to the "reframing [of] both the moral and biological content of the condition [severe mental illness]"; and in ways that would have beneficially challenged the "habits of mind" of Republican-era readers (Gibson & Jacobson 2018, p. 187).

Politics and the press in greater China

Although culturally Chinese communities, the political differences across mainland China, Hong Kong, and Taiwan are stark. The Communist Party has ruled mainland China since 1949, following the defeat of the Nationalist Party forces. While economic and social policy on the mainland over the past seven decades has vacillated from extreme leftist orthodoxy to market-based socialism, the authority of the Communist Party, notionally representing the democratic voice of the masses, has remained supreme and unchallenged. This continues to the present day, where political orthodoxy, albeit far from leftist, holds sway. While Hong Kong returned to the People's Republic of China in 1997 as a special administrative region, it retains a high degree of local autonomy in the running of its day-to-day affairs. The local executive body, ExCo [行政會議], does so under the oversight of the local legislative body, Legco [立法會]. These local bodies, nevertheless, work under a putative constraint that rule of the People's Republic of China by the Communist Party is supreme and not to be questioned in any way. Taiwan, by contrast, has essentially functioned as a liberal democracy since the late 1980s, after the disbanding of the Nationalist Party dictatorship. This dictatorship had ruled the island from 1949, when the Nationalist Party forces fled the mainland, following their defeat by the Communists.

The Communist Party forthrightly controls the mainland Chinese press. As stated in the Chapter 2 section on the Chinese-language newspapers, the *People's Daily* is the official messenger of the party (Brady 2002; Cao 2014; Lee 2015; Yang & Parrott 2018). As such, it sets the political tone for reporting on any issue of substance on the mainland (Sandby-Thomas 2014). The multitude of regional and sectional newspapers across mainland China dutifully follow its lead. Failing to do so would bring sanction. This regulatory role of the *People's Daily* is backed up by a well-developed state apparatus for media control and censorship (Brady 2008). Ultimate power lies in the hands of the Central Propaganda Department of the Communist Party (Brady 2008). It even controls and censors media reports on health topics (Brady 2008, 2012). Accordingly, the *People's Daily* reporting on matters such as current government policy on severe mental illness strictly adheres to the dictates of the party and the state. As the official messenger of the party, reporting of this type is common in the newspaper. Numerically, political reports rank second only to medical reports in the *People's Daily* corpus (see Chapter 2 section on the news reports). By contrast, the number of political reports in the *Ming Pao* and *Liberty Times* corpora is extremely low.

Although now a part of the People's Republic of China, media controls in Hong Kong are considerably more lax than those on the mainland. Local newspapers regularly present a range of viewpoints and takes on issues, as they do in Asian democracies such as Japan, Singapore, and Taiwan. There is no omnipresent state oversight of the media in Hong Kong, like that on the mainland. Local newspapers, nevertheless, tend to be careful not to cross the political line concerning the sovereignty of the People's Republic of China and supreme rule by the Communist Party. Doing so might attract the wrath of the central authorities in Beijing. Newspapers in Taiwan, of course, are free from such concerns. Yet, like their Hong Kong counterparts, their political reporting is often shaped by the stance of the media organisation to which they belong, as opposed to that of the ruling party. The section on the Chinese-language newspapers in Chapter 2 outlines the broad political stances of *Ming Pao* and *Liberty Times*.

Political reports

The *People's Daily* reports on political issues in, and current government policy on, severe mental illness focus on the social and legal management of those with the illness; as well as improving health service affordability and delivery in rural and remote areas. The former issue positively calls attention to the control the party and state have over an illness that can threaten the mainland's valued social harmony and social stability. The latter issue is a policy rallying point of the national government at present. These *People's Daily* reports typically describe government policy on severe mental illness and its wider mental health strategy, in an uncritical way. There is no reporting of the opinion of mental health activists of any kind. The reports do not cluster in any month or in any section of the newspaper (see Appendix 1). This means that, across an extended twelve-month period of analysis, there is regular, consistent, positive reporting on government policy on severe mental illness and its wider mental health strategy.

By contrast, their *Ming Pao* and *Liberty Times* counterparts report on the opinions of local mental health activists, the former much more so than the latter. They also cluster in particular months, unlike the *People's Daily* reports. The *Ming Pao* reports cluster in April and May of 2016, while those in *Liberty Times* cluster in March and April of 2016 (see Appendices 2 and 3). The *Ming Pao* cluster coincides with a spate of leading public figures in Hong Kong, including local politicians and academics, making defamatory figurative statements about people with a severe mental illness. In response, local people with the illness and their supporters called for Hong Kong society to resolutely tackle such blatant discrimination against those with the illness. The *Liberty Times* cluster, on the other hand, coincides with the random brutal killing of a young girl on a street in Taipei in late March 2016. Although the mental health status of her murderer had not yet been officially ascertained, the local police implied that he was suffering from a severe mental illness at the time of the killing. Most of these *Ming Pao* and *Liberty Times* reports appear in the newspapers' local news sections (see Appendices 2 and 3). Publishing in the most-read section of the newspaper would give them greater prominence.

Nearly all of the political reports in all three Chinese-language newspapers deal with generic severe mental illness (see Appendices 1–3). For the *Liberty Times*, this contrasts with its reports from the other thematic categories, which uniformly focus on depression. Georgaca and Bilić (2007) state that reporting on generic severe mental illness, rather than on specific diagnostic categories such as depression, discursively homogenises those with the illness. Doing so makes it easier to mark them out as a "deviant" other, who "exist as an imagined community living somewhere" removed from everyday society, namely, hidden inside their family home or in a prison-like psychiatric facility (Guo 2016, p. 2). This appears to be particularly advantageous in the political domain.

The *People's Daily* political reports name severe mental illness in this generic way at the uppermost level of the news text superstructural hierarchy. In doing so, the headlines not only discursively homogenise people with a severe mental illness, but they also nominally reduce them to the status of "sufferer/patient" (see selected Examples 11 and 12).

11　Concern Over Dispersal Of <u>Mental Illness Sufferers</u> – How To Resolve This? [精神病人散落之忧如何解] (#15)

12　Taking Care Of <u>Mental Illness Sufferers</u> – Society Must Not Be "Lax" [照护精神病患，社会别"大撒把"] (#17)

Example 11 initially casts those with a severe mental illness, in a homogenising and stigmatising way, as an emerging problem for mainland Chinese society. Those who are now problematically being "dispersed" in everyday society, by corollary, would have previously lived apart from this society, in line with Chinese cultural stigma. A question about how to take care of this problem immediately follows the initial claim. Doing so militates against any interrogation of the stigmatic premise on which this claim is based. The headline maintains focus on people with a severe illness by concealing, through nominalisation, any other social actors in play, namely, those who are concerned, those who are dispersing people with the illness, and those who are set to resolve the problem. Example 12 similarly maintains attention on those with a severe mental illness by grammatically concealing who is "taking care of" them, and generically naming all others as "society." The headline also maintains an authoritarian, institutional tone through its use of the command modal "must." Other headlines do so through their use of imperative clauses that voice the demands of those in positions of political power (see selected Example 13).

13　<u>National People's Congress Representative Wu Xiangdong</u>: <u>Pay Attention To</u> Psychological Health Of Nation's People [全国人大代表吴向东: 关注国民心理健康] (#9)

No headlines of the *People's Daily* political reports give people with a severe mental illness agency. They remain voiceless as others disperse or take care of them. The headlines of their *Liberty Times* counterparts similarly deny those with the illness agency, even in activist reports (see selected Examples 14 and 15).

14　<u>Forcibly Put</u> "Shaky Bro" In Hospital – <u>KP</u> Attacked For <u>Trampling On</u> Human Rights [强制「摇摇哥」送醫 柯P被轟踐踏人權] (#132)

15　<u>Police Float</u> Killer Mentally Ill – <u>Doctor Forthrightly Says</u> Too Arbitrary [警定調兇手是精障 醫師直言太武斷] (#138)

Example 14 gives agency to the mayor of Taipei, locally dubbed "KP," who "tramples on" the human rights of a well-known local homeless man, "Shaky Bro," by "forcibly" hospitalising him. Shaky Bro has a chronic severe mental illness. The use of the passive voice, "attacked," further conceals the identities of those who advocate on Shaky Bro's behalf, retaining focus on the person in authority. Example 15 similarly gives voice to those in authority, namely, the "police," but also gives voice to an advocate for the person with a severe mental illness. The example, however, names the advocate not by his personal name but by his authoritative professional status: "a doctor." It further nominally links severe mental illness to extreme violence, "killing," in line with prevailing stigmatic attitudes and beliefs. The headlines of conventional, non-activist *Liberty Times* political reports, in like manner, explicitly link severe mental illness to criminal violence (see selected Examples 16 and 17).

16 Homicide, Correctional Rehabilitation & Psychopathology [殺人、教化與精神病理] (#112)
17 Child Killer Suspect Mentally Ill? Politician Criticises Criminal Investigation Division, Fears Will Help Killer Get Off [殺童嫌精神病？議員批刑大恐幫脫罪] (#135)

The headlines of the *Ming Pao* political reports, by contrast, never link severe mental illness to criminality of any kind, despite the newspaper's thematic predilection for doing so (see Chapter 3 section on crime reports). Instead, the reports give greater agency to people with a severe mental illness by naming them by their personal names, or naming them collectively, but not by way of their illness (see selected Examples 18–20).

18 People In Recovery: Social Environment Is More Troublesome [康復者：社會環境更困擾] (#47)
19 People With Personal Experience Make Declaration – Hope To Eliminate Misunderstanding About Severe Mental Illness – Resent "Ravings, Weird Behaviour" Remarks By Chris Wat Wing-Yin – Plan To File Complaint With Equal Opportunities Commission [過來人親身發聲冀消除精神病誤解 不滿屈穎妍「妄語怪行」論 擬平機會投訴] (#48)
20 Vincent Cheng: Let's Rise Up Against Remarks Defaming Mentally Ill! [鄭仲仁：我們就來起義，反對抹黑精神病人的言論！] (#57)

These headlines further give voice to activist statements and "declarations" by people with a severe mental illness, which, in empowering ways, displace blame away from themselves and onto wider Hong Kong society; and assert their self-determination to "eliminate," "resent," "plan," "complain," and "rise up."

The *People's Daily* and *Liberty Times* political reports spell out how people with a severe mental illness are a problem to the wider society in the reporting beyond the headline. This reporting in both newspapers points to the "propensity for violence" [有暴力倾向] and "aggression" [攻擊性] of those with the illness, at this upper level of the news text superstructural hierarchy. They are "ticking time bombs" [不定時炸彈], who often commit "atrocities" [慘劇] that are disturbingly "indiscriminate" [素不相识], "inexplicable" [莫名其妙], and "completely unpredictable" [完全不可预测]. Moreover, their crimes are "recurrent" [不时/ 再次/ 一一幕] and "bizarre" [匪夷所思] and, so, "continually attract the attention of the general public" [始终没离开公众视野]. In this way, the reports transfigure the subjectivity of those with a severe mental illness from that of a reductive biomedical "sufferer" [病患/ 病人/ 患者] to that of an impersonal, legalistic "case" [案], "criminal suspect" [兇嫌], "murderer" [殺人犯/ 兇手], "latent killer" [潛在還沒犯下死罪的人], and "one who is at risk of harming others" [傷人之虞]. The *Liberty Times* reports notably epitomise this in the man who randomly decapitated a young girl on the streets of Taipei. They consistently topicalise him in the opening clauses of the opening paragraphs of their news stories. Such casting of those with a severe mental illness as a social threat justifies their rigorous supervision and control by those in authority. Government agencies "observe" [觀察], "identify" [鑑定/ 認定], "assess" [評估], "handle" [處理], and "manage" [管理] them. Restrictive biomedical "measures" [措施], such as "involuntary hospitalisation" [強制送醫/ 強制住院] and "involuntary treatment" [強制就醫/ 強制治療], facilitate this in Taiwan. Their *People's Daily* counterparts, on the other hand, disclose how the mainland Chinese state marks out those with a severe mental illness as a discrete social "group" [群体], whose members are systematically tracked on a "national register" [全国登记在册]. This is because they can be violent and "hinder social productivity and improvement in the people's level of happiness" [阻碍了社会生产力和人民幸福水平的提升]. As such, they work against the state's primary political agenda of maintaining social harmony and social stability, and improving the living standards of everyday citizens.

By contrast, the *Ming Pao* political reports detail how contemporary Hong Kong society continues to stigmatise people with a severe mental illness, at this upper level of the news text superstructural hierarchy. In doing so, they identify the wider society as the primary problem rather than those with the illness. They point to how leading local public figures needlessly and cruelly deride "worthless youth" [廢青], who recently had taken part in Hong Kong independence demonstrations, as "a pack of mental illness sufferers" [一群精神病人], who "must be strictly controlled to prevent harm to society" [必須嚴厲控制，以防危害社會]. Other public figures, in turn, criticise these stigmatic conflations that denigrate those with a severe mental illness. Despite this singularly activist sentiment of the *Ming Pao* political reports, they seldom give voice to those with the illness at this upper level of the news text superstructural hierarchy. Those in authority largely speak on their behalf.

This silencing of people with a severe mental illness in the *Ming Pao* political reports continues into the lower levels of the news text superstructural hierarchy, despite their activist tone. More sensitive naming of those with the illness, too, is relegated to the lower levels of the discursive hierarchy. Labels include:

- "service consumer" [服務消費者].
- "person with life experience" [生活經歷者].
- "client" [客戶].
- "person who has experienced severe mental illness" [精神病過來人].

- "person with a psychiatric diagnosis" [有精神科診斷的人士].
- "person with a mental disorder" [有精神障礙的人士].

At the lower levels of the news text superstructural hierarchy, the *Liberty Times* and *People's Daily* political reports, on the other hand, pose a solution to the key problem identified earlier on in the news story, namely, that people with a severe mental illness present a threat to everyday society. People in authority invariably pose these solutions. The solutions that they pose consistently strengthen governmental oversight of and control over those with the illness. This manifests, in disempowering ways, through enhanced public security measures, forced hospitalisation of those with the illness, and the ratification of legislation that expressly limits their human rights as compared to mentally well citizens (see selected Examples 21–24).

21 First, the state should consider amending the Mental Health Act and significantly increase content that deals with mental-health-related statutes. Second, improve the quality of specialised education in psychology, supporting growth in the study of basic psychology and applied psychology, thus encouraging more high-quality young people to devote themselves to this cause of great social value. Third, increase the strength of publicity about mental health. Fourth, fully incorporate psychological treatment into the scope of medical care and insurance. [第一，国家应该考虑修订《精神卫生法》，大幅增加心理健康相关的法规内容；第二，提升心理学专业教育的质量，支持基础心理学和应用心理学的发展，鼓励更多高素质的年轻人投身到这个有巨大社会价值的事业中；第三，加大心理健康的宣传力度；第四，把"心理治疗"全面纳入医保范围。] (#9)

22 Second, improve the communication and coordination mechanism. The task of compulsory treatment involves multiple agencies, such as public security, state prosecutors [the "procuratorate"], courts, and compulsory treatment bodies. It also involves different departments within the procuratorial office. In order to strengthen the all-round, timely, and effective control of this task, it is suggested that every local political and legal committee take the lead and formulate practical and feasible means for implementation; and establish a mechanism for improving linkages and communication, together with a mechanism for information networking. This will boost cooperation and coordination between public security, the procuratorate, courts, and compulsory treatment bodies, and lay a solid foundation for the legal supervision of the implementation of compulsory treatment. [二、健全沟通协作机制。强制医疗工作涉及公安、检察、法院及强制医疗机构等多个主体，还涉及检察机关内部的不同部门。为了加强对此项工作全面、及时、有效的监督，建议由各地政法委牵头，制定切实可行的实施办法，建立健全衔接沟通机制和信息联网机制，促进公安、检察、法院及强制医疗机构之间的协作配合，为强制医疗执行法律监督工作奠定坚实基础。] (#10)

23   The psychological or psychopathological condition of murderers at the time of their crime are tasks for judicial psychiatric evaluation, and also important points of reference for prosecution and sentencing. [殺人犯案發當時的精神狀態與精神病理，是司法精神鑑定的工作，也是起訴與量刑的重要參考。] (#112)

24   Ting Chih-Wei, a psychiatrist at the Nanshih branch of Da Chien General Hospital, said that some people who are suspected of having psychiatric symptoms lack insight into their illness and, so, obstructively refuse medical treatment. When they do not meet the criteria for forced hospitalisation, their families and related units can only advise them or quietly put up with them. Sufferers who have previously received medical treatment, yet who often are unwilling to return for their regular outpatient treatment, can be medically examined and treated at home by specialist psychiatric treatment staff at set times. This provides professional medical treatment and, so, reduces the number of cases of relapse. [大千綜合醫院南勢分院精神科醫師丁志偉表示，疑似精神症狀者，礙於本身沒有病識感而不願意就醫，又未達強制住院的標準，家屬及相關單位只能勸說或隱忍，而曾接受治療的患者，也常不願意定期回門診就醫，居家治療是由精神科醫療專業人員定期到府看診，提供專業醫療、減少個案疾病再發。] (#133)

Examples 21 and 22 from the *People's Daily* speak in an institutional way, using enumerated lists, nominalisation, and passive voice (Ramsay 2008). Example 21 topicalises the "state" as the prime agent from the outset. Thereafter, it maintains the agency of the state by grammatically obscuring that of others, through nominalisations such as "education," "growth," "study," "publicity," "treatment," "care," and "insurance." It also blurs the boundaries between biomedicine and the law, through the lexical conjoining of "mental health" to "acts" and "statutes," and through advancing "psychology" as a "cause of great social value" and, so, political value to the state. In like manner, a heavily nominalised Example 22 legalistically links the involuntary treatment of people with a severe mental illness to "public security, the procuratorate, courts, and compulsory treatment bodies." It also similarly gives agency to state-sponsored "political and legal committees," which actively and positively "take the lead," formulate," "establish," "boost," and "lay a solid foundation." Doing so allows the mainland Chinese state to successfully "control," in a paternalistic way, people with a severe mental illness, to the betterment of society.

Examples 23 and 24 from *Liberty Times* also blur the boundaries between biomedicine and the law, but with greater problematising of people with a severe mental illness as a danger to society. Example 23 lexically conjoins "psychiatry" to the "judiciary," who "evaluate," "refer," "prosecute," and "sentence" those with the illness, in like manner to Example 21. However, Example 23 further forensically links "psychopathology" to "murder," in a threatening way. In like manner, Example 24 prioritises the authoritative voice of the health professional, in legalistically casting those with "psychiatric symptoms" as "suspects." Moreover, they not only lack the insight of the knowledgeable health professional, but actively resist and frustrate her or his attempts to help them. The example further depersonalises them, in institutional and culturally stigmatic ways, as "cases" subject to "criteria" that others can use to legally remove them from everyday society. Their cultural status as non-persons is additionally borne out by their families having "to put up with them"; and their apparent "unwillingness" to abide by schedules that are "set" by "specialist psychiatric treatment staff," who merely want to help them and prevent them from "relapsing" into an undesirable state of personhood.

In sum, governing authorities cast severe mental illness as a pressing social problem in the *People's Daily* and *Liberty Times* political reports, from the uppermost levels of their news text superstructural hierarchy. The government, reassuringly, can credibly solve this problem, by systematically supervising and controlling those with the illness. This may entail removing them from everyday society, in line with long-standing Chinese cultural stigma (Guo 2016; Kleinman, Yan, Jun et al. 2011; Ramsay 2013; Wang & Liu 2016; Zhuang, Wong, Cheng et al. 2017). The ability of those in authority to solve this problem bears out a broader political agenda in mainland China and Taiwan. By removing the threat posed by those with a severe mental illness, in particular, their proclivity for violence, mainland Chinese authorities fulfil their long-standing, primary political commitment to maintain social harmony and social stability. The *People's Daily* reporting of this type is consistent over time. While necessarily at the expense of people with the illness, such reporting aligns with the long-standing Chinese cultural stigma that casts them as wholly disruptive and undesirable. By contrast, such reporting is sporadic and clustered in *Liberty Times*. The authorities in Taiwan, seemingly, only react following publicly contentious acts of random violence by those with a severe mental illness. This points to a more reactive political, and electoral, imperative to protect mentally well citizens from harm, rather than ongoing validation of a leading ideological tenet.

While society is the victim of the threat posed by severe mental illness in the *People's Daily* and *Liberty Times* political reports, it is cast as the stigmatic villain in their *Ming Pao* counterparts. As a result, they are decidedly more activist in tone. They call attention to the stark challenges that people with a severe mental illness face in their day-to-day lives. They also redirect blame for these challenges away from people with the illness and onto wider society. In addition, they prioritise the voice of those with the illness at the uppermost level of the superstructural hierarchy. Despite these empowering features, the voice of authority dominates the penultimate and lowest levels of the superstructural hierarchy. The authorities regularly depersonalise those with the illness by naming them using reductive biomedical and institutional labels, as their *People's Daily* and *Liberty Times* counterparts do. This occurs regardless of whether the authority is a conservative politician or a liberal activist. The empowerment expressed in the *Ming Pao* political reports is further tempered by their concomitant casting of society as a stigmatic villain and a principal source of support for people with a severe mental illness. Just like their *People's Daily* and *Liberty Times* counterparts, they cast society as a place that people with the illness should aspire to return to in a productive capacity. This is in line with the dominant cultural narrative in collectivist Chinese societies (Ramsay 2013, 2016). As a result, people with a severe mental illness are directed to return to a place that relentlessly subjugates and marginalises them. Similar contradictions also mark Chinese life stories, filmic stories, and literary stories of severe mental illness (Linder 2011; Ramsay 2013; Rojas 2011).

The establishment and severe mental illness

The analysis shows how elite narratives of the orthodox biomedical and political establishments appear to direct and shape the medical reports and political reports in the three Chinese-language newspapers. This is mostly to the detriment of people with a severe mental illness. The impact of the salience of these narratives on lay readers' "habits of mind" in relation to the illness would likely be greatest in mainland China (Gibson & Jacobson 2018, p. 187). This is because the biomedical reports and political reports account for more than half of the reports in the *People's Daily* corpus. By comparison, they only account for around a quarter of the reports in the *Ming Pao* and *Liberty Times* corpora.

The reports on current medical findings about severe mental illness and related disorders, such as prevalence rates, causes, early warning signs, and treatments, as well as available support services and public health measures, bear out and endorse an orthodox biomedical narrative that preferentially locates knowledge and power in the hands of health professionals; causally sequences the lived experience of severe mental illness by way of the clinical paradigm of symptoms > diagnosis > treatment; places heavy value on medically supervised treatment, in particular, pharmacotherapy; and depersonalises people with a severe mental illness by subjectively reducing them to their illness or related clinical entity. The medical reports lack Mishler's (1984, p. 104) emblematic "voice of the lifeworld." They silence the voice of those with the illness, with those in authority speaking on their behalf. This maintains the cultural status quo in mainland China, Hong Kong, and Taiwan, whereby laypeople defer to the professional opinions and expert status of those in authority (Ng 2000; Ramsay 2008, 2013; Shi-xu 2014; Zhuang, Wong, Cheng et al. 2017). This also maintains the cultural status quo that stigmatically casts people with a severe mental illness as voiceless non-persons (Guo 2016; Kleinman, Yan, Jun et al. 2011; Rosenberg 2018; Wu 2010).

In like manner, the *People's Daily* and *Liberty Times* reports on political issues in, and current government policy on, severe mental illness bear out and endorse primary narratives of governance in mainland China and Taiwan, respectively. These narratives confirm the authoritative role of the government in severe mental illness, regardless of political system. The authority of the governments of mainland China and Taiwan over this illness stems from the laws of their lands. The *People's Daily* and *Liberty Times* political reports regularly point out that governing authorities can, and should, legally compel those with the illness to take medication, or legally remove them from everyday society and into prison-like psychiatric facilities (Angermeyer & Schulze 2001; Blood, Putnis, & Pirkis 2002; Clement & Foster 2008). This is because they can be prone to violent acts. As such, the governments of mainland China and Taiwan are merely acting to protect their mentally well citizens in accordance with the law. This blurs the boundaries between biomedicine and the law. Remedial biomedical responses are undistinguishably predicated upon the law. Reporting in this way exploits severe mental illness for political gain. The mainland Chinese government demonstrates that it can successfully maintain social harmony and social stability, a long-standing political tenet of the Open Door reform period (Brady 2008, 2009; Cao 2014; Choy 2016; Sandby-Thomas 2014). The Taiwan government demonstrates that it can guarantee the personal safety of its citizens. This likely is of electoral value to the ruling party. Such reporting also maintains the cultural status quo in mainland China and Taiwan, whereby people with a severe mental illness are stigmatically cast as a social threat that must be removed (Guo 2016; Kleinman, Yan, Jun et al. 2011; Ramsay 2013).

By contrast, the *Ming Pao* political reports, while small in number, bear out and endorse a more activist narrative that promotes the human rights of those with a severe mental illness. Such reporting would be expected to challenge the political and cultural status quos in Hong Kong, by humanising those with the illness and casting them as equals to their mentally well compatriots. However, this apparent empowerment of those with the illness is concomitantly offset by the silencing of their voice. Others continue to speak on their behalf. As such, the *Ming Pao* political reports cede power to those in authority, as the political reports in the other two newspapers do. Moreover, even though the *Ming Pao* political reports cast society as a villain, an equal number of its *medical* reports cast society as a victim, as the *People's Daily* and *Liberty Times* political reports and medical reports do. As a result, the activist sentiment in the *Ming Pao* political reports is offset by the culturally more orthodox sentiment in its medical reports.

The analysis finds that both categories of reports in all three newspapers consistently bear out and endorse a culturally aligned return-to-society script in severe mental illness. This narrative, in a disempowering way, measures people's recovery from illness by their ability to productively contribute to their families and the wider society, in line with long-standing Chinese cultural scripts (Jacka 2014; Ramsay 2013, 2016). Baum (2018) historically traces the authoritative linking of "mental rehabilitation with labor and economic viability" to Republican-era China where, "[b]efore a lunatic was released from the asylum, he was often made to promise that he would henceforth engage in productive work" (p. 52). Then, as now, social productivity was clearly gendered in line with normative femininity and masculinity (Jacka 2014; Ramsay 2013, 2016), with women with a severe mental illness "not expected to make such a claim, though their return to a domestic setting likely implied a similar outcome" (Baum 2018, p. 52). The return-to-society script is problematic for people with a severe mental illness, as very few of them likely can regain the required levels of social functioning. Their failure to do so, in turn, confirms the cultural status quo that stigmatically casts them as not just disruptive but socially undesirable (Guo 2016; Kleinman, Yan, Jun et al. 2011; Ramsay 2013). The narrative is equally problematic in compelling them to return to the same society that likely made them ill and marks them out as a non-person.

Cao (2014) states that, "[a]s an authoritarian society, political discourse" in mainland China "carries the highest order of importance and, despite the substantial retreat of politics from people's lives in the post-reform era, still has a pervasive impact upon all aspects of society" (p. 2). This means that the greater salience of the elite narratives of the orthodox biomedical and political establishments in the *People's Daily* reports has political import and is socially purposeful. The reports document how the government looks to science, namely, orthodox biomedicine, to solve the problem of severe mental illness. Science is highly credible (Fairclough 2003; Georgaca & Bilić 2007; van Leeuwen 2007; Whitley & Hickling 2007). It also is a fundamental tenet of Marxism and the ideology of the Chinese Communist Party in the Open Door reform period (Bakken 2000; Brady 2002, 2009; Lin 2017). As such, the government's systematic response to severe mental illness is both rational and politically correct. What is more, the orthodox biomedical narrative justifies the state's pharmacotherapeutic management and remedial control of those with the illness, including their removal from everyday society into prison-like psychiatric facilities. This, in turn, converges with the state's primary political narrative of the Open Door reform period, namely, maintenance of social harmony and social stability above all on the mainland. In effect, the elite orthodox biomedical narrative is co-opted to bolster the elite political narrative. In this way, the mainland Chinese state can legitimately direct and manage its citizens, while masking any control that it concurrently gains over them.

This concomitant masking of state control as remedial care and therapeutic management in the *People's Daily* medical reports and political reports also calls attention to the government's infallible, benevolent, constructive role in severe mental illness. It commendably provides protective legislation and wide-ranging healthcare services and subsidies that target those with the illness. Their families and wider society may fail them (Guo 2016), but the infallible state never does. Moreover, the state's paternalistic control over those with a severe mental illness benefits the entire nation (Shi-xu 2014), by pharmacotherapeutically correcting members of a "deviant" community (Guo 2016, p. 2), who, consequently, can return to society in a productive capacity. Those members who cannot be corrected, such as violent *"wu fengzi"*

[武疯子] (Guo 2016, p. 203), are safely removed from everyday society, into psychiatric facilities. This, as always, is in accordance with the law.

The blurring of the boundaries between biomedicine and the law sets these news reports apart from their Western counterparts. While the orthodox voice of biomedicine often colonises the latter (Dubugras, Evans-Lacko, & de Jesus 2011; Georgaca & Bilić 2007; Harper 2009; Rowe, Tilbury, Rapley et al. 2003), doing so operates more as "a strategy for destigmatising mental 'breakdown'," as "just another illness anyone can 'get'." That is to say, severe mental illness is just like any commonplace physical illness, such as diabetes, asthma, or hypertension. Doctors can readily treat it. By contrast, the *People's Daily* medical reports and political reports appear to purposely co-opt the orthodox voice of biomedicine, in order to legitimise the mainland Chinese state's paternalistic control over its citizens (Rowe, Tilbury, Rapley et al. 2003, p. 692). The smaller in number *Liberty Times* counterparts also do so in like manner, paying greater attention to the needs of the collective, namely, society, at the expense of the individual. This occurs even though it is a largely liberal leaning newspaper. The converse generally holds for the more activist *Ming Pao* political reports, but not for its medical reports. Analogous Western reporting is similarly equivocal, but with greater individualistic inclinations (Yang & Parrott 2018; Zhang, Jin, & Tang 2015).

References

Angermeyer, M. C., & Schulze, B. (2001). Reinforcing stereotypes: How the focus on forensic cases in news reporting may influence public attitudes towards the mentally ill. *International Journal of Law and Psychiatry, 24*(4), 469–486.

Bakken, B. (2000). *The exemplary society: Human improvement, social control, and the dangers of modernity in China*. Oxford: Oxford University Press.

Baum, E. (2018). *The invention of madness: State, society, and the insane in modern China*. Chicago: University of Chicago Press.

Blood, R. W., Putnis, P., & Pirkis, J. (2002). Mental-illness news as violence: A news frame analysis of the reporting and portrayal of mental health and illness in Australian media. *Australian Journal of Communication, 29*(2), 59–82.

Brady, A. (2000). Treat insiders and outsiders differently: The use and control of foreigners in the PRC. *The China Quarterly, 164*(2000), 943–964.

Brady, A. (2002). Regimenting the public mind: The modernization of propaganda in the PRC. *International Journal, 57*(4), 563–578.

Brady, A. (2008). *Marketing dictatorship: Propaganda and thought work in contemporary China*. Lanham, MD: Rowman & Littlefield.

Brady, A. (2009). Mass persuasion as a means of legitimation and China's popular authoritarianism. *American Behavioral Scientist, 53*(3), 434–457.

Brady, A. (2012). State Confucianism, Chineseness, and tradition in CCP propaganda. In A. Brady (Ed.), *China's thought management* (pp. 57-75). London: Routledge.

Cao, Q. (2014). Introduction: Legitimisation, resistance and discursive struggles in contemporary China. In Q. Cao, H. Tian, & P. A. Chilton (Eds.), *Discourse, politics and media in contemporary China* (pp.1–24). Amsterdam: John Benjamins.

Choy, H. Y. F. (2016). Introduction: Disease and discourse. In H. Y. F. Choy (Ed.), *Discourses of disease: Writing illness, the mind and the body in modern China* (pp. 1–15). Leiden: Brill.

Clement, S., & Foster, N. (2008). Newspaper reporting on schizophrenia: A content analysis of five national newspapers at two time points. *Schizophrenia Research, 98*(1), 178–183.

Dubugras, M. T. B., Evans-Lacko, S., & de Jesus Mari, J. (2011). A two-year cross-sectional study on the information about schizophrenia divulged by a prestigious daily newspaper. *The Journal of Nervous and Mental Disease, 199*(9), 659–665.

Every-Palmer, S., Brink, J., Chern, T. P., Choi, W. K., Hern-Yee, J. G., Green, B., Heffernan, E., Johnson, S. B., Kachaeva, M., Shiina, A., Walker, D., Wu, K., Wang, X., & Mellsop, G. (2014). Review of psychiatric services to mentally disordered offenders around the Pacific Rim. *Asia-Pacific Psychiatry, 6*(1), 1–17.

Fairclough, N. (2003). *Analysing discourse: Textual analysis for social research.* New York: Routledge.

Georgaca, E., & Bilić, B. (2007). Representations of "mental illness" in Serbian newspapers: A critical discourse analysis. *Qualitative Research in Psychology, 4*(1), 167–186.

Gibson, C., & Jacobson, T. (2018). Habits of mind in an uncertain information world. *Reference and User Services Quarterly, 57*(3), 183–192.

Guo, J. (2016). *Stigma: An ethnography of mental illness and HIV/AIDS in China.* Hackensack, NJ: World Century.

Harper, S. (2009). *Madness, power and the media: Class, gender and race in popular representations of mental distress.* Basingstoke, UK: Palgrave Macmillan.

Jacka, T. (2014). Left-behind and vulnerable? Conceptualising development and older women's agency in rural China. *Asian Studies Review, 38*(2), 186–204.

Kleinman, A., Yan, Y., Jun, J., Lee, S., Zhang, E., Pan, T., Wu, F., & Guo, J. (2011). *Deep China: The moral life of the person: What anthropology and psychiatry tell us about China today.* Berkeley, CA: University of California Press.

Lee, H. W. (2015). From control to competition: A comparative study of the party press and popular press. In G. D. Rawnsley & M. T. Rawnsley (Eds.), *Routledge handbook of Chinese media* (pp. 117–130). New York: Routledge.

Li, G., Gutheil, T. G., & Hu, Z. (2016). Comparative study of forensic psychiatric system between China and America. *International Journal of Law and Psychiatry, 47*(2016), 164–170.

Lin, D. (2017). Civilising citizens in post-Mao China: Understanding the rhetoric of *suzhi*. New York: Routledge.

Linder, B. (2011). Trauma and truth: Representations of madness in Chinese literature. *Journal of Medical Humanities, 32*(4), 291–303.

Maggs, E. (2012). *A cultural analysis of suicide in the Chinese classical novels* Romance of the Three Kingdoms *and* Dream of Red Mansion [BA Honours dissertation, The University of Queensland].

Ministry of Health and Welfare. (2017). *Taiwan health and welfare report 2017.* Taipei: Ministry of Health and Welfare, R.O.C. (Taiwan).

Mishler, E. G. (1984). *The discourse of medicine: Dialectics of medical interviews.* Norwood: Ablex.

Ng, R. M. (2000). The influence of Confucianism on Chinese conceptions of power, authority, and the rule of law. In D. R. Heisey (Ed.), *Chinese perspectives in rhetoric and communication* (pp. 45–56). Stamford: Ablex.

Patel, V., Xiao, S., Chen, H., Hanna, F., Jotheeswaran, A. T., Luo, D., Parikh, R., Sharma, E., Usmani, S., Yu, Y., Druss, B. G., & Saxena, S. (2016). The magnitude of and health system responses to the mental health treatment gap in adults in India and China. *The Lancet, 388*(10063), 3074–3084.

Phillips, M., Chen, H., Diesfeld, K., Xie, B., Cheng, H., Mellsop, G., & Liu, X. (2013). China's new mental health law: Reframing involuntary treatment. *American Journal of Psychiatry, 170*(6), 588–591.

Ramsay, G. (2008). *Shaping minds: A discourse analysis of Chinese-language community mental health literature.* Amsterdam: John Benjamins.

Ramsay, G. (2013). *Mental illness, dementia and family in China.* London: Routledge.

Ramsay, G. (2016). *Chinese stories of drug addiction: Beyond the opium dens.* New York: Routledge.

Rojas, C. (2011). Of canons and cannibalism: A psycho-immunological reading of "Diary of a Madman." *Modern Chinese Literature and Culture, 23*(1), 47–76.

Rosenberg, A. (2018, 18 June). Hiding my mental illness from my Asian family almost killed me: The silent shame of having a mental illness in a Chinese family. *Vox.* www.vox.com/first-person/2018/6/18/17464574/asian-chinese-community-mental-health-illness

Rowe, R., Tilbury, F., Rapley, M., & O'Ferrall, I. (2003). "About a year before the breakdown I was having symptoms": Sadness, pathology and the Australian newspaper media. *Sociology of Health and Illness, 25*(6), 680–696.

Sandby-Thomas, P. (2014). "Stability overwhelms everything": Analysing the legitimating effect of the stability discourse since 1989. In Q. Cao, H. Tian, & P. A. Chilton (Eds.), *Discourse, politics and media in contemporary China* (pp. 47–76). Amsterdam: John Benjamins.

Shi-xu. (2014). *Chinese discourse studies.* Hampshire, UK: Palgrave Macmillan.

Topiwala, A., Wang, X., & Fazel, S. (2012). Chinese forensic psychiatry and its wider implications. *Journal of Forensic Psychiatry and Psychology, 23*(1), 1–6.

van Leeuwen, T. (2007). Legitimation in discourse and communication. *Discourse and Communication, 1*(1), 91–112.

Whitley, R., & Hickling, F. W. (2007). Open papers, open minds? Media representations of psychiatric de-institutionalization in Jamaica. *Transcultural Psychiatry, 44*(4), 659–671.

World Health Organization. (2011). *Mental health atlas 2011: China, Hong Kong Special Administrative Region.* Geneva: Department of Mental Health and Substance Abuse, World Health Organization.

World Health Organization. (2014). *Mental health atlas 2014: China.* Geneva: Department of Mental Health and Substance Abuse, World Health Organization.

Wu, F. (2010). *Suicide and justice: A Chinese perspective.* New York: Routledge.

Xu, X., Li, X. M., Xu, D., & Wang, W. (2017). Psychiatric and mental health nursing in China: Past, present and future. *Archives of Psychiatric Nursing, 31*(5), 470–476.

Xue, L., Shi, Y. W., Knoll, J., & Zhao, H. (2015). Chinese forensic psychiatry: History, development and challenges. *Journal of Forensic Science and Medicine, 1*(1), 61–67.

Yang, Y., & Parrott, S. (2018). Schizophrenia in Chinese and U.S. online news media: Exploring cultural influence on the mediated portrayal of schizophrenia. *Health Communication, 33*(5), 553–561.

Zhang, Y., Jin, Y., & Tang, Y. (2015). Framing depression: Cultural and organizational influences on coverage of a public health threat and attribution of responsibilities in Chinese news media, 2000–2012. *Journalism and Mass Communication Quarterly, 92*(1), 99–120.

Zhuang, X. Y., Wong, D. F. K., Cheng, C. W., & Pan, S. M. (2017). Mental health literacy, stigma and perception of causation of mental illness among Chinese people in Taiwan. *International Journal of Social Psychiatry, 63*(6), 498–507.

6 Conclusion
Reporting mental illness in China

Newspaper reporting can significantly shape how people make sense of severe mental illness (Kesic, Ducat, & Thomas 2012; Ma 2017; Nairn, Coverdale, & Coverdale 2011; Peng & Tang 2010; Rukavina, Nawka, Brborović et al. 2012; Thornicroft, Goulden, Shefer et al. 2013; Whitley & Berry 2013; Whitley & Wang 2017; Zhang, Jin, & Tang 2015). It may draw on prevailing narratives, confirm them, legitimise them, or challenge them. The analyses in Chapters 3, 4, and 5 identify discursive features and strategic trends in the reporting on severe mental illness in three leading Chinese-language broadsheet newspapers from mainland China, Hong Kong, and Taiwan. These features and trends variably stem from a report's naming and gendering practices; designation of causation and blame; affirmation of explanatory models; the granting of voice and agency; and selective othering of those with the illness. The overall arrangement, distribution, and frequency of the features and trends bear out dominant cultural, political, and biomedical narratives that circulate in a geographical community. These narratives cast those with a severe mental illness, their family caregivers, their health professionals, and others in authority in ways that are familiar to the wider society. The prevailing narratives in culturally Chinese communities severely stigmatise those with the illness (Guo 2016; Ramsay 2008, 2013). As a result, effective counter-narratives should aim to uniquely humanise, include, and empower them.

The social transgressor

The *Ming Pao* and *Liberty Times* reports regularly cast people with a severe mental illness as social transgressors and, most threateningly, violent criminals. Doing so links them to disdained social outgroups that most citizens would want to rid from everyday society (Richardson 2007; van Dijk 2000, 2014, 2015). Severe mental illness seemingly breeds, attracts, or incites social transgression and criminality. Fifty-three percent of *Ming Pao* reports on the illness and 40% of their *Liberty Times* counterparts cast it in this way. As such, the two newspapers devote quite a large amount of print space to detrimental reporting that confirms and legitimises long-standing stigmatic cultural attitudes and beliefs, namely, that people with the illness should be feared. The *Ming Pao* reports heighten this fear by focusing more often on violent crime and calling attention to the apparent randomness of such crime. Any everyday citizen could be the next victim. By contrast, the *Liberty Times* reports magnanimously give greater attention to people with a severe mental illness who are the victims of crime. This more closely approaches the reality of their experience of crime (Cashman & Thomas 2017; Hsu, Sheu, Liu et al. 2009; Rukavina, Nawka, Brborović et al. 2012; Varshney, Mahapatra, Krishnan et al. 2016). Despite this greater magnanimity of the *Liberty Times* reports, they, like their *Ming Pao* and *People's Daily* counterparts, commonly deny those with the illness any agency beyond their perpetrating of socially transgressive acts. The *Liberty Times* reports additionally cast women with the illness as morally and sexually suspect. The mentally ill women may be victims of crime, but they often intimately know the men who perpetrate these crimes against them. This deflects some of the blame for the crimes onto the women victims. At the same time, this confirms and legitimises a prevailing detrimental gender narrative that contends that women often attract such crime (Burnett, Mattern, Herakova et al. 2009; Cowan 2000; Suarez & Gadalla 2010).

Reporting on crime and social wrongdoing in sensational ways sells newspapers. This is obviously important in commercial media markets such as Hong Kong and Taiwan. Western newspapers do the same (Angermeyer & Schulze 2001; Olstead 2002; Richardson 2007). Reporting in this way, however, only enhances the prevailing fear of people with a severe mental illness as dangerous social threats. As such, they should be removed from everyday society, just as common criminals are, and just as long-standing Chinese cultural scripts dictate. This way they can do no harm to society.

The triumphant man and fruitless woman

Telling life stories about everyday people's experiences of an illness gives insight that more authoritative state, institutional, and biomedical accounts lack (Brody 2003; Bury 2001; Charon 2006; Frank 1995; Garden 2010; Hydén 1997; Kleinman 1988; Thomas 2010). Severe mental illness is no exception. *Ming Pao* and *Liberty Times* acknowledge, at least to a limited degree, the value of everyday people's life stories, with just over one in ten reports recounting such stories. By contrast, the *People's Daily* seemingly dismisses their value, due to the absence of reporting on them over an extended twelve-month period of analysis. They evidently serve no social or political purpose for this messenger of the Communist party and the mainland Chinese state.

Although *Ming Pao* and *Liberty Times* recount life stories of everyday people with a severe mental illness, authoritative others generally narrate these stories. The voice of everyday people with the illness, accordingly, is diminished. It seems that those with the illness lack the credibility or, even, the right to speak. The reporting in all three newspapers further diminishes the life stories of everyday people with the illness by recounting those of celebrities in equal or greater measure. The celebrity life stories that are recounted equate to inspirational testimony or sensational tattletale. Inspirational testimonies recount how celebrities with a severe mental illness, usually men, successfully overcome their illness through their own efforts, and return to society in a productive capacity. In this way, they regain their socially ascribed personhood that those with a severe mental illness lack, according to long-standing stigmatic cultural attitudes and beliefs. By contrast, women celebrities either overcome their illness with the help of others, usually men, or fail to overcome their illness and socially transgress, often in quite salacious ways. This is especially so in the *People's Daily* reporting, where all the women celebrities are from, and continue to reside in, Hong Kong, Taiwan, and Singapore. Reporting on the salacious behaviour of local women celebrities would contravene current media prohibitions against the reporting of celebrity tattletale on the mainland (Shepherd 2017).

The *Ming Pao* and *Liberty Times* reports gender everyday people's life stories of severe mental illness in like manner. Everyday men with the illness, once again, singularly overcome their illness and return to society in a productive capacity. They also magnanimously share their story of success, most likely in the hope of inspiring others with the illness to do likewise. By contrast, everyday women with the illness overcome their illness with the help of others in the *Liberty Times* reports, or they fail to do so in their *Ming Pao* counterparts. The women who overcome their illness in the *Liberty Times* reports additionally exhibit their new-found social success by way of their culturally normative feminine achievements as wives, mothers, and daughters.

The underrepresentation of women in success narratives about severe mental illness in all three Chinese-language newspapers bears out exemplary norms and scripts in Chinese culture (Jacka 2014; Roberts 2014). Men more plausibly overcome adversity in exemplary ways, while women fail to do so. The suicide reports in all three newspapers are gendered in similar ways. In these reports, women with a severe mental illness more frequently commit ignominious suicide, even though men with the illness, in reality, do so with equal or greater frequency across greater China (see Chapter 3 section on suicide in present-day greater China). It appears to be less culturally confronting for a woman with the illness to commit ignominious suicide, given that being a woman, as well as having severe mental illness, traditionally are subordinate states of being in Chinese culture.

The patient

The *People's Daily* reports are distinct in uniformly casting people with a severe mental illness as objects of medical attention, namely, patients, regardless of thematic category. By contrast, *Ming Pao* and *Liberty Times* largely limit this to their medical reports. These reports account for a much lower proportion of their newspaper corpora than their *People's Daily* counterparts. The latter reports further consistently augment the difference between healthy people and mentally ill patients, by naming the latter using reductive generic labels rather than specific diagnostic classifications (Georgaca & Bilić 2007). Marking out patients in this homogenising way justifies the mainland Chinese state's sweeping legislative and policy responses to severe mental illness. This is because they are clearly targeted at a discrete social group that can cause problems for everyday citizens. Moreover, the state's management and control of this group has a legal mandate and, so, is just and humane.

The *People's Daily* reports necessarily subordinate the voice of the patients to that of authoritative experts, namely, government officials and health professionals. The latter's voice depersonalises patients as objects to be acted upon. The state and allied health professionals work hand in hand to systematically count, monitor, examine, regulate, and experiment on their bodies. Doing so blurs the disciplinary boundaries between biomedicine and the law, placing power to manage and control these people in the hands of the paternalistic state. The state has the interests of all citizens at heart: both mentally ill patients and the mentally well. Casting those with a severe mental illness in this way adds weight to Zhang, Jin, and Tang's (2015, p. 111) claim that newspaper reporting on the mainland commonly renders those with the illness "invisible." The focus, instead, is steadfastly placed on the nation (Shi-xu 2014). This maintains time-honoured political and social status quos on the mainland, where social harmony, social stability, and social control are paramount, and the needs and rights of the many far outweigh those of the few (Choy 2016; Shi-xu 2014; Zhang, Jin, & Tang 2015).

The reporting in the three Chinese-language newspapers, therefore, casts patients somewhat differently, depending on their pragmatic intention. Orthodox biomedicine helps patients recover, in the *Ming Pao* and *Liberty Times* reports. As a result, they no longer are at risk of being social threats, who may harm everyday citizens on occasion. In like manner, health professionals seek to help patients, by monitoring them and ensuring that they are pharmacotherapeutically compliant. This is world's best practice medicine. By contrast, the *People's Daily* reports cast the benevolent state as the primary agent of oversight of patients, and their strict management and control. To do so, the state strategically co-opts orthodox biomedicine, in a rational and scientific way, to systematically ensure the ongoing safety of the nation and, so, maintain social harmony and social stability. As such, these reports impersonally construct severe mental illness as an objective clinical category rather than a subjective life experience. Mishler's (1984, p. 104) emblematic "voice of the lifeworld," accordingly, is nowhere to be found.

The (unspeakably) monstrous schizophrenic

The reporting in all three Chinese-language newspapers exhibits a stigmatic hierarchy of severe mental illness, according to diagnostic label. Schizophrenia consistently holds the uppermost position in this stigmatic hierarchy. The construction of schizophrenia as the most disturbing and confounding of severe mental illnesses in the reporting in the three newspapers aligns with long-standing stigmatic attitudes and beliefs in culturally Chinese communities (Pearson 1996; Ramsay 2008, 2013; Tang & Bie 2015). The illness is widely disdained because it violates cultural norms and values that laud social and familial harmony, and productive contribution to society and the family (Jacka 2014). The reporting in the *People's Daily* illustratively warns that schizophrenia is "the most serious kind of mental illness" [精神类疾病中最严重的一种], which can cause those with the illness to suffer "irreversible brain damage" [大脑神经会发生不可逆的损伤]. It further cautions that those with the illness have a proclivity to "reduce or stop using medication on their own accord" [自行减药或停止用药], even though "pharmacotherapy is the most important form of treatment" [药物治疗是最主要的治疗方法]. The reporting in *Ming Pao* and *Liberty Times* similarly counsels that legislated compulsory pharmacotherapy is essential if governments wish to effectively address the problem of schizophrenia.

While the reporting in all three newspapers consistently casts schizophrenia as the most monstrous of severe mental illnesses, how it does so differs from newspaper to newspaper. The reporting in *Ming Pao* appears to exploit the negative reputation of the illness, by over-reporting on it relative to its prevalence in the local community. The prevalence is around 0.4 per hundred people across greater China, as well as Western countries such as Australia and the Netherlands (Charlson, Ferrari, Santomauro et al. 2018). The reporting in *Ming Pao* additionally homes in on sensationally transgressive events where schizophrenia is at issue, such as violent crime. Doing so taps into the prevailing social fear of people with schizophrenia as unpredictable and dangerous. The reporting in *Liberty Times*, on the other hand, numerically aligns with the prevalence of the illness in the community. While the reporting does not appear to numerically exploit the negative reputation of the illness in the sensational way that the *Ming Pao* reporting does, there is a common topical focus on violent crime, and biomedical-cum-legal means to manage and control those with the illness. By contrast, the *People's Daily* rarely reports on the illness. It seemingly avoids reporting on an unspeakable illness that the wider community so disdains (Tang & Bie 2015). Reporting on it as *Ming Pao* and *Liberty Times* do would likely be of little social or political benefit to the mainland Chinese state.

The infallible state

The reporting on severe mental illness in the *People's Daily* is distinct from its *Ming Pao* and *Liberty Times* counterparts, due to its greater, consistent focus on the nation rather than the illness or people with the illness. Regardless of the topic of a news text, it calls attention to the role of the state in managing and controlling the vexed social issue of severe mental illness. The state's actions are uniformly rational and justified, because they are grounded in contemporary science, namely, orthodox biomedicine. They also are invariably successful. They, nevertheless, are neatly circumscribed in the reports. The state can readily intervene in most domains of social life, except within the family. As a result, on the comparatively rare occasions that the reports deal with crime or social wrongdoing, they attribute any blame for the transgressions committed by those with a severe mental illness to parents. The state necessarily mops up the consequences of such parental failures. Moreover, as with all matters related to severe mental illness on the mainland, the state response necessitates enforcing strict social management and control, using available corrective, legislative, and pharmacotherapeutic means.

Accordingly, the wider narratives about severe mental illness that emerge from the *People's Daily* reports are highly consistent, evidenced based, and nation centred. Moreover, they usefully align with leading contemporary political narratives that extol the virtues of social harmony, social stability, and the rule of law on the mainland. In this way, the reports effectively make use of severe mental illness to corroborate and validate these primary political tenets. Even with a social concern as troublesome and complex as severe mental illness, the benevolent, infallible state is clearly well prepared and well equipped to credibly, appropriately, justly, humanely, and efficaciously respond nationwide, to the betterment of mentally ill and mentally well citizens alike. These existing political and emergent media narratives conveniently align with long-standing stigmatic attitudes and beliefs in Chinese culture that people with a severe mental illness should be removed from everyday society, confined to the family home, or detained in secure institutions (Baum 2018; Ramsay 2013). In the case of the *People's Daily*, the state is the agent of these necessary actions that are carried out with unerring success and in line with world's best medical practices.

Nascent tensions and contradictions

These discursive constructions and their attendant narratives contribute to nascent tensions and contradictions in the reporting on severe mental illness in all three Chinese-language newspapers. These include apparent paradoxes and mismatches within the content of what is reported; between what is reported and generic conventions and expectations; as well as between what is reported and social reality.

Paradoxes and mismatches within the content of what is reported over the periods of analysis include the magnanimous naming of severe mental illness, while casting it in highly detrimental ways. The reporting in *Ming Pao* and *Liberty Times* regularly names schizophrenia using the neutral neologism *sijueshitiao* [思覺失調]. Doing so responds, in a positive way, to the intense cultural stigma that accompanies the conventional diagnostic label *jingshenfenlie* [精神分裂] (see Chapter 1 section on news media reporting of mental illness in greater China). Despite this, the reporting continues to cast schizophrenia in highly detrimental ways, and deny those with the illness any voice, even when they are a celebrity. The greater use of the neutral neologism in the

Ming Pao reports corroborates Chan, Ching, Lam et al.'s (2017) claim that Hong Kong newspapers preferentially use this label to denote schizophrenia and related psychoses. The regular use of the label in the *Ming Pao* reporting on violent crime where perpetrators have schizophrenia, however, refutes their claim that Hong Kong newspapers tend to revert to the conventional diagnostic label when reporting on such crime. Guo (2016) and Kleinman, Yan, Jun et al. (2011) point out that the stigmatic othering and dehumanisation of people with schizophrenia in culturally Chinese communities facilitate their removal from everyday society into prison-like psychiatric facilities and, less commonly but more dreadfully, their existential erasure from their families through mercy killing.

The reporting in all three Chinese-language newspapers on crime where severe mental illness is implicated contradictorily casts those with the illness as both "mad" and "rational" (Olstead 2002, p. 630). While seemingly insane, they carry out (criminal) acts that require elements of thought and planning. Olstead (2002) identifies a similar contradiction in Western reporting on the illness. Equally contradictory, *Ming Pao*, arguably the most sensational of the three newspapers, reports most on social and political activism in severe mental illness. This occurs even though most of its reporting on the illness validates, rather than counters, long-standing cultural stigma against the illness. By contrast, *Liberty Times*, arguably the most magnanimous of the three newspapers, reports comparatively less on social and political activism in severe mental illness. In addition, it places greater responsibility on families to care for those with the illness, in line with traditional cultural practices and expectations (Baum 2018). Current legislation in Taiwan and mainland China does likewise (Chou 2006; Every-Palmer, Brink, Chern et al. 2014; Li, Gutheil, & Hu 2016; Phillips, Chen, Diesfeld et al. 2013; Topiwala, Wang, & Fazel 2012; Xue, Shi, Knoll et al. 2015). The apparent magnanimity of the *Liberty Times* reporting is also at odds with its readiness to fall back on the stigmatic cultural stereotype of the violent mentally ill criminal, following the random brutal killing of a young girl on the streets of Taipei by a man whose mental health status was yet to be determined. It seems that this negative stereotype is never far from mind.

There is additional mismatch between the reporting of everyday people's life stories of severe mental illness in *Ming Pao* and *Liberty Times*, and wider narrative conventions and expectations. A doctor-centred orthodox voice of biomedicine consistently colonises these life stories, even though one may anticipate greater resonance of Mishler's (1984, p. 104) emblematic "voice of the lifeworld." This colonisation by the orthodox voice of biomedicine likely stems from family caregivers telling the life stories, rather than people with the illness. The former appear to have greater narrative credibility in severe mental illness. A similar discursive phenomenon marks life stories of severe mental illness that are told by family caregivers for psychoeducational purposes in mainland China. I analyse these life stories in Ramsay (2013). I find that Chinese cultural norms, values, and scripts, and a desire to retain a degree of social face, likely shape these stories in this way. Specifically, the family caregivers are

i   socially "one step removed from the illness" (Ramsay 2013, p. 58), since they are not the person with the illness, who can be stigmatically marked and reductively defined by the language of orthodox biomedicine, such as "diagnosis," "prognosis," "case," and "schizophrenia."
ii well versed in the biomedical explanatory model of severe mental illness, due to regular coaching by treating health professionals. Chinese cultural norms, values, and scripts compel laypeople to accede to the advice and direction of those in authority with specialist knowledge (Ng 2000; Ramsay 2008, 2013; Shi-xu 2014; Zhuang, Wong, Cheng et al. 2017). By publicly doing so, the family caregivers can gain a degree of face.
iii implicitly seeking to make others aware of their solid commitment to orthodox biomedical reasoning, thereby affirming their wholehearted commitment to restoring the health of their ill family member. This is their cultural duty.

The resulting silence of people with severe mental illness in the life stories reported in *Ming Pao* and *Liberty Times* is not only disempowering for them, but it also detrimentally amplifies and consolidates their social otherness and lack of personhood. Accordingly, readers' "habits of mind" in relation to the illness remain unchallenged and unchanged (Gibson & Jacobson 2018, p. 187).

Paradoxes and mismatches between what is reported and social reality include the most stigmatic reporting on severe mental illness occurring in the geographical community where factual knowledge about it is greatest, namely, Hong Kong. *The Ming Pao* reporting seemingly prioritises sensationalism and, so, commercial sales, over community psychoeducation. Hui, Tang, Wong et al. (2013), nevertheless, point to the greater success of community psychoeducation in Hong Kong, when compared to mainland China and Taiwan. Chen, Wu, and Huang (2014, p. 440) tellingly calculate that as many as "40% of people with schizophrenia and their families" in Taiwan "believ[e] that the cause of schizophrenia was related to the supernatural phenomenon." Similar thinking about severe mental illness has permeated the mainland since traditional times to date (Baum 2018; Chen, Wu, & Huang 2014; Hui, Tang, Wong et al. 2013; Li & Phillips 1990; Ran, Xiang, Simpson et al. 2005; Yip 2007). It, therefore, is a somewhat constructive development that the reporting in the *People's Daily* and *Liberty Times* tends to sensationalise the illness less and biomedicalise it more, albeit in orthodox ways that endorse its management and control by those in authority.

All three newspapers exhibit a clear mismatch between the frequency with which they report on suicide by women with a severe mental illness, and the gendered reality for suicide incidence. They over-report on women's suicide, when men commit suicide to an equal or greater degree across greater China (see Chapter 3 section on suicide in present-day greater China). This gendered incidence for suicide is common across the globe (Galasiński 2013, 2017; Sun & Zhang 2017; Wang, Chan, & Yip 2014). The greater coverage of women's suicide in the three Chinese-language newspapers likely stems from its sensational and, so, commercial, value; as well as it being less culturally confronting than ignominious suicide by men. This is because women traditionally have a subordinate status in Chinese culture.

The reporting in all three newspapers also paradoxically advocates that people demonstrate their recovery from a severe mental illness by successfully returning to everyday society in a productive capacity. This rigidly compels them to return to the same society that stigmatises them so severely, unsympathetically, and relentlessly; and likely contributed to their illness in the first place. The reporting lacks more realistic, nuanced, person-centred definitions of recovery, despite the widely recognised diversity of people's experience of severe mental illness across the globe.

Chinese versus Western news reporting on severe mental illness

The analyses in Chapters 3 to 5 reveal ostensible similarities and differences between the reporting on severe mental illness in the three Chinese-language newspapers and that in Western counterparts. They further show that problematic reporting often stems from quite different discursive practices and forces, many of which are cultural in origin (Shi-xu 2014, 2015).

The reporting in the three Chinese-language newspapers prioritises the voice of those in authority over that of people with a severe mental illness, as many Western counterparts do. Those in authority include health professionals, government officials, politicians, academics, and the police. Their voices are deemed credible. Prioritising their voice over that of people with the illness, however, is widely recognised to be problematic in the West (Ramsay 2008; Rowe, Tilbury, Rapley et al. 2003). Accordingly, media reporting now tends to give greater attention to a variety of voices, including those of people with the illness. By contrast, prioritising the voice of those in authority is not problematic in culturally Chinese communities. Doing so accords with persuasive norms in Chinese culture that esteem and place high standing on specialist knowledge and professional expertise (Ng 2000; Ramsay 2008; Shi-xu 2014; Zhuang, Wong, Cheng et al. 2017). As a result, Chinese readers would expect that newspaper reporting on social phenomena like severe mental illness prioritises the voice of those in authority.

The reporting in the Chinese-language newspapers also prejudicially genders severe mental illness in detrimental ways. Western reporting commonly casts men with a severe mental illness as "fundamentally 'bad'," while women with the illness are fundamentally "sad" (Whitley, Adeponle, & Miller 2015, p. 331). Although both states of being are decidedly negative, the bad mentally ill men gain greater agency. They act singularly and volitionally, albeit irrationally. The reporting in the Chinese-language newspapers also gives greater agency to men, especially those with depression, and more often in positive and constructive ways that align with masculine norms in Chinese culture. In this way, these men can serve as social exemplars in severe mental illness. By contrast, Galasiński (2008, p. 121) finds that, in Poland, men's depression

> is invariably constructed as an assault on masculinity – the social expectations of what it means to be a man, what a man does (or should do), his role at work, in the family and so on [...] On the one hand, it undermines masculinity, depressed men are not men, or at the very least are lesser men. On the other hand, depression disturbs masculinity, it makes it impossible to execute it.

Women with a severe mental illness rarely serve as social exemplars in the reporting in the three Chinese-language newspapers. They more commonly violate feminine norms in Chinese culture, and only overcome their illness with the help of others. This selective, gendered empowerment of men may stem, once again, from womanhood and severe mental illness traditionally being subordinate conditions in Chinese culture. As a result, men more commonly serve as social exemplars, while women less problematically fail (Jacka 2014; Roberts 2014).

The reporting in the Chinese-language newspapers locates severe mental illness in a stigmatic hierarchy, according to diagnostic label. Western reporting also does, detrimentally linking diagnostic label to socioeconomic class and, in turn, race (Harper 2009; Olstead 2002). The "socially connected" middle classes, who tend to be white, commonly have depression, an illness readily associated with overextension and exhaustion (Olstead 2002, p. 640). By contrast, the socially ostracised poorer classes, who tend to be non-white, commonly have schizophrenia, an illness readily associated with illicit drug abuse (Olstead 2002). A negative social outcome of reporting in this way is that depression and, so, white people, receive more economic resources and support from those in authority. By contrast, the stigmatic hierarchy in the reporting in the Chinese-language newspapers stems less from class and race and more from long-standing cultural norms, values, and scripts. These norms, values, and scripts cast schizophrenia as the most disturbing of severe mental illnesses (Pearson 1996; Ramsay 2013; Tang & Bie 2015).

Van Dijk (2000) lists a series of discursive strategies that Western newspapers and like media use to invalidate and discredit social others, such as new migrants and refugees. These include:

1 Delegitimating membership: they do not belong here, in our group, in our country in our city, in our neighbourhood, in our organization.
2 Delegitimating actions, including discourse: they have no right to engage in what they do or say, for example work here, or accuse us of racism; criminalization of actions (e.g. "illegal entry").

3 Delegitimating goals: they only come here to take advantage of our welfare system.

4 Delegitimating norms and values: their values are not ours; they should adapt to our culture; we are not used to that here.

5 Delegitimating social position: for example, they are not real refugees, but merely economic ("fake") ones.

(van Dijk 2000, p. 259)

Similar strategies mark the reporting on severe mental illness in the three Chinese-language newspapers. It regularly casts those with the illness as menacing non-persons, in line with Chinese cultural stigma (Guo 2016; Kleinman, Yan, Jun et al. 2011). They are "deeply disturbing within Chinese society" (Pearson 1996, p. 438). They have irrepressibly different norms, values, and behaviours that trouble everyday citizens. They frequently transgress, often in criminal ways. They also are unproductive and, so, an economic burden on their family, society, and the nation as a whole. As a result, they deserve no social rights or voice, since they are not "a normal person with social face and dignity" (Guo 2016, p. 31). They further do not belong in everyday society. Instead, they should be confined to the family home or incarcerated in prison-like psychiatric facilities (Baum 2018). Here, they are safely removed from everyday society. This is not inhumane, as they are not real people with real lives.

Towards a more compassionate, inclusive, humane, and empowering construction of severe mental illness in newspaper reporting across greater China

The Chapter 1 section on Chinese discourse studies on mental illness shows how a wide range of texts drawn from the present-day and the past – official pronouncements, psychoeducational brochures, personal life stories, films and literary works – construct mental illness in ways that marginalise, disempower, and dehumanise people with the illness, in line with long-standing cultural stigma. The analyses in Chapters 2 to 5 identify similar trends in the reporting in the three Chinese-language newspapers from greater China. At the same time, the analyses implicitly and explicitly point to pathways to more compassionate, inclusive, and humanising reporting on severe mental illness in greater China, which constructively empowers and minimises difference (Bhui & Bhugra 2002; Dixon-Woods 2001; Fleischman 2003; Harper 1996).

Liberty Times exhibits more traces of magnanimous reporting than the *People's Daily* and *Ming Pao*. The broadsheet newspaper from Taiwan reports comparatively less on crime where people with a severe mental illness are the perpetrators, and more on crime where they are victims. This aligns more with the social reality of the illness (Cashman & Thomas 2017; Hsu, Sheu, Liu et al. 2009; Rukavina, Nawka, Brborović et al. 2012; Varshney, Mahapatra, Krishnan et al. 2016). The newspaper also defers disclosure of the mental health status of perpetrators and victims of crime to subordinate levels of the news text superstructural hierarchy. This tempers the oft-made link between severe mental illness and violence. The newspaper additionally confers greater diversity on the experience of the illness, by regularly differentiating diagnostic categories. It further assigns diagnostic labels to those with the illness in ways that do not reductively essentialise their subjectivities. This militates against homogenisation of the experience, which readily facilitates social othering (Georgaca & Bilić 2007; Knifton & Quinn 2008; Wahl, Wood, & Richards 2002). The newspaper draws greater attention to mitigating aetiological factors and forces in severe mental illness, which are beyond the immediate control of those with the illness. This redirects blame (or cause) away from them, and onto the wider society, the environment, or biomedicine (Tolton 2009).

All three newspapers silence the voice of people with a severe mental illness. Their silence only amplifies and consolidates their other-ness and lack of personhood. While Chinese culture values the voice of authority, there is cultural precedence for recounting the voice of laypeople (Lu 2000; Qiu 2000; Wang 2002; Shi-xu 2014). Doing so enhances authenticity and normalises diversity in the experience of severe mental illness. Anonymity would need to be maintained if reporting of this type were to be pursued. This is because public disclosure of severe mental illness in culturally Chinese communities risks great loss of face by those with the illness, as well as their family members (Guo 2016; Ramsay 2008, 2013; Rosenberg 2018; Tang & Bie 2015). A high degree of journalistic expertise and insight would be crucial. As Whitley, Adeponle, and Miller (2015) caution, news "stories about mental illness per se appear to be more positive and less stigmatizing than articles focused upon individuals identified as having a real or alleged mental illness" (p. 330). This is

> because generic articles are often in-depth well-researched longer pieces written by a specialist health journalist. In contrast, articles about an individual [...] are often written by general journalists with little knowledge of health or mental health issues per se.
>
> (Whitley, Adeponle, & Miller 2015, pp. 330–331)

The findings of this book also point to the need for greater attention to gender in newspaper reporting on severe mental illness across greater China. The reported experiences of men and women with the illness should be more nuanced and well rounded, reflecting the diversity of what happens in reality. The voice of mental health activists, while controversial, can further complement that of laypeople with a severe mental illness. *Ming Pao* and *Liberty Times* only sporadically report on activist sentiment, and only in reaction to a recent local incident. More conspicuously, the *People's Daily* never does, since doing so may bring the authority of the infallible state into question. Yet, only through regular newspaper reporting of the nuanced and diverse voices of laypeople and mental health activists can a much-needed compassionate, inclusive, humane, and empowering counter-narrative of severe mental illness come to pass and, so, beneficially challenge readers' "habits of mind" in relation to the illness (Gibson & Jacobson 2018, p. 187).

Conclusion

Nairn (2007, p. 143) states that "the intertextuality of madness [...] both maintains and elaborates accumulated meanings of madness across a variety of texts and media." *Reporting Mental Illness* finds that newspaper reporting across greater China often validates the stigmatic casting of people with a severe mental illness as "deviant individuals" in Chinese culture (Guo 2016, p. 2). Such reporting can only "sustain and reproduce the social status quo," rather than contest and counter it (Angermuller, Maingueneau, & Wodak 2014, p. 362. See also Tian 2012; Wang 2015). The book, however, finds that the reporting is not relentlessly negative, in contrast to the writing and depictions in Chinese-language texts from other genres, such as literary works and films, even those by progressive authors and artists.

The book points out ways in which newspaper reporting on severe mental illness can create a more magnanimous counter-narrative that contests prevailing social, cultural, and political status quos across greater China. These status quos currently dehumanise, marginalise, and disempower those with the illness. Developing such a counter-narrative, however, is not an easy task. This is because commercial pressures in the media encourage sensationalist reporting. Newspaper reporting on severe mental illness also is very resistant to change over time (Kesic, Ducat, & Thomas 2012; McGinty, Kennedy-Hendricks, Choksy et al. 2016; Nairn, Coverdale, & Coverdale 2011; Rhydderch, Krooupa, Shefer et al. 2016). Baum (2018) tellingly points out in her cultural history of early twentieth-century China that

> Throughout the early republic, the print media often presented madness as violent, salacious, and obscene. In tabloids, mad people yelled and cursed, disemboweled themselves and slit their own throats, disrobed in the streets and caused public commotions. They were, at best, objects of public fascination and, at worst, targets of public disgust.
>
> (p. 97)

Such reporting is reminiscent of that in *Ming Pao* today.

The pace of recasting media narratives about severe mental illness cannot exceed a readership's readiness to accept them. Entrenched Chinese cultural imaginings and positionings constitute profound impediments to any such change. What is more, substantial shift in social, cultural, and political status quos requires attention on all generic fronts, not just on news texts (Anderson 2003; Chilton, Tian, & Wodak 2012; Nairn 2007; Olstead 2002; Reisigl & Wodak 2009; Richardson 2007). A holistic response is required yet, seemingly, far from reach at present.

Greater China accounts for around one-fifth of the world's population. Mainland China, alone has the largest number of people with a severe mental illness in the world. People from greater China also make up large immigrant groups in many Western countries. Mental health agencies in these countries are increasingly looking to evidence bases to inform their approaches to mental health delivery, in increasingly culturally diverse clinical settings. This book contributes to such evidence bases. In doing so, it hopes to inform wider attempts and endeavours to humanise, include, and empower people with a severe mental illness, across greater China and the global Chinese diaspora.

References

Anderson, M. (2003). "One flew over the psychiatric unit": Mental illness and the media. *Journal of Psychiatric and Mental Health Nursing, 10*(3), 297–306.

Angermeyer, M. C., & Schulze, B. (2001). Reinforcing stereotypes: How the focus on forensic cases in news reporting may influence public attitudes towards the mentally ill. *International Journal of Law and Psychiatry, 24*(4), 469–486.

Angermuller, J., Maingueneau, D., & Wodak, R. (2014). Critical approaches: Introduction. In J. Angermuller, D. Maingueneau, & R. Wodak (Eds.), *Discourse Studies reader: Main currents in theory and analysis* (pp. 359–364). Amsterdam: John Benjamins.

Baum, E. (2018). *The invention of madness: State, society, and the insane in modern China*. Chicago: University of Chicago Press.

Bhui, K., & Bhugra, D. (2002). Explanatory models for mental distress: Implications for clinical practice and research. *The British Journal of Psychiatry, 181*(1), 6–7.

Brody, H. (2003). *Stories of sickness*. Oxford: Oxford University Press.

Burnett, A., Mattern, J. L., Herakova, L. L., Kahl, D. H. Jr., Tobola, C., & Bornsen. S. E. (2009). Communicating/muting date rape: A co-cultural theoretical analysis of communication factors related to rape culture on a college campus. *Journal of Applied Communication Research, 37*(4), 465–485.

Bury, M. (2001). Illness narratives: Fact or fiction? *Sociology of Health and Illness, 23*(3), 263–285.

Cashman E. L., & Thomas. S. D. M. (2017). Does mental illness impact the incidence of crime and victimisation among young people? *Psychiatry, Psychology and Law, 24*(1), 33–46.

Chan, S. K. W., Ching, E. Y. N., Lam, K. S. C., So, H., Hui, C. L. M., Lee, E. H. M., Chang, W. C., & Chen, E. Y. H. (2017). Newspaper coverage of mental illness in Hong Kong between 2002 and 2012: Impact of introduction of a new Chinese name of psychosis. *Early Intervention in Psychiatry, 11*(4), 342–344.

Charlson, F. J., Ferrari, A. J., Santomauro, D. F., Diminic, S., Stockings, E., Scott, J. G., McGrath, J. J., & Whiteford, H. A. (2018). Global epidemiology and burden of schizophrenia: Findings from the Global Burden of Disease Study 2016. *Schizophrenia Bulletin, 44*(6), 1195–1203.

Charon, R. (2006). *Narrative medicine: Honoring the stories of illness*. Oxford: Oxford University Press.

Chen, F., Wu, H., & Huang, C. (2014). Influences of attribution and stigma on working relationships with providers practicing Western psychiatry in the Taiwanese context. *Psychiatric Quarterly, 85*(4), 439–451.

Chilton, P., Tian, H., & Wodak, R. (2012). Reflections on discourse and critique in China and the West. In P. Chilton, H. Tian, & R. Wodak (Eds.), *Discourse and socio-political transformations in contemporary China* (pp. 1–18). Amsterdam: John Benjamins.

Chou, J. Y. (2006). *The psychiatric politics of risk and cost: Forensic theory and practice in the US and Taiwan.* [Doctoral dissertation, Seattle, WA: University of Washington].

Choy, H. Y. F. (2016). Introduction: Disease and discourse. In H. Y. F. Choy (Ed.), *Discourses of disease: Writing illness, the mind and the body in modern China* (pp. 1–15). Leiden: Brill.

Cowan, G. (2000). Women's hostility toward women and rape and sexual harassment myths. *Violence against Women, 6*(3), 238–246.

Dixon-Woods, M. (2001). Writing wrongs? An analysis of published discourses about the use of patient information leaflets. *Social Science and Medicine, 52*(9), 1417–1432.

Every-Palmer, S., Brink, J., Chern, T. P., Choi, W. K., Hern-Yee, J. G., Green, B., Heffernan, E., Johnson, S. B., Kachaeva, M., Shiina, A., Walker, D., Wu, K., Wang, X., & Mellsop, G. (2014). Review of psychiatric services to mentally disordered offenders around the Pacific Rim. *Asia-Pacific Psychiatry, 6*(1), 1–17.

Fleischman, S. (2003). Language and medicine. In D. Schiffrin, D. Tannen, & H. E. Hamilton (Eds.), *The handbook of discourse analysis* (pp. 470–502). Oxford: Blackwell.

Frank, A. W. (1995). *The wounded storyteller: Body, illness, and ethics.* Chicago: University of Chicago Press.

Galasiński, D. (2008). *Men's discourses of depression.* London: Palgrave Macmillan.

Galasiński, D. (2013). *Fathers, fatherhood and mental illness: A discourse analysis of rejection.* London: Palgrave Macmillan.

Galasiński, D. (2017). *Discourses of men's suicide notes: A qualitative analysis.* New York: Bloomsbury Academic.

Garden, R. (2010). Telling stories about illness and disability: The limits and lessons of narrative. *Perspectives in Biology and Medicine, 53*(1), 121–135.

Georgaca, E., & Bilić, B. (2007). Representations of "mental illness" in Serbian newspapers: A critical discourse analysis. *Qualitative Research in Psychology, 4*(1), 167–186.

Gibson, C., & Jacobson, T. (2018). Habits of mind in an uncertain information world. *Reference and User Services Quarterly, 57*(3), 183–192.

Guo, J. (2016). *Stigma: An ethnography of mental illness and HIV/AIDS in China.* Hackensack, NJ: World Century.

Harper, D. J. (1996). Deconstructing "paranoia": Towards a discursive understanding of apparently unwarranted suspicion. *Theory and Psychology, 6*(3), 423–448.

Harper, S. (2009). *Madness, power and the media: Class, gender and race in popular representations of mental distress.* Basingstoke, UK: Palgrave Macmillan.

Hsu, C. C., Sheu, C. J., Liu, S. I., Sun, Y. W., Wu, S. I., & Lin, Y. (2009). Crime victimization of persons with severe mental illness in Taiwan. *Australasian Psychiatry, 43*(5), 460–466.

Hui, C., Tang, L., Wong, M., Chang, J., Chan, Y., Lee, G., & Chen, H. (2013). Predictors of help-seeking duration in adult-onset psychosis in Hong Kong. *Social Psychiatry and Psychiatric Epidemiology, 48*(11), 1819–1828.

Hydén, L. C. (1997). Illness and narrative. *Sociology of Health and Illness, 19*(1), 48–69.

Jacka, T. (2014). Left-behind and vulnerable? Conceptualising development and older women's agency in rural China. *Asian Studies Review* , *38*(2), 186–204.

Kesic, D., Ducat, L. V., & Thomas, S. D. (2012). Using force: Australian newspaper depictions of contacts between the police and persons experiencing mental illness. *Australian Psychologist, 47*(4), 213–223.

Kleinman, A. (1988). *The illness narratives: Suffering, healing, and the human condition.* New York: Basic Books.

Kleinman, A., Yan, Y., Jun, J., Lee, S., Zhang, E., Pan, T., Wu, F., & Guo, J. (2011). *Deep China: The moral life of the person: What anthropology and psychiatry tell us about China today.* Berkeley, CA: University of California Press.

Knifton, L., & Quinn, N. (2008). Media, mental health and discrimination: A frame of reference for understanding reporting trends. *International Journal of Mental Health Promotion, 10*(1), 23–31.

Li, G., Gutheil, T. G., & Hu, Z. (2016). Comparative study of forensic psychiatric system between China and America. *International Journal of Law and Psychiatry, 47*(2016), 164–170.

Li, S., & Phillips, M. R. (1990). Witch doctors and mental illness in mainland China: A preliminary study. *The American Journal of Psychiatry, 147*(2), 221–224.

Lu, X. (2000). The influence of classical Chinese rhetoric on contemporary Chinese political communication and social relations. In D. R. Heisey (Ed.), *Chinese perspectives in rhetoric and communication* (pp. 3–24). Stamford: Ablex.

Ma, Z. (2017). How the media cover mental illnesses: A review. *Health Education, 117*(1), 90–109.

McGinty, E. E., Kennedy-Hendricks, A., Choksy, S., & Barry, C. L. (2016). Trends in news media coverage of mental illness in the United States: 1995–2014. *Health Affairs, 35*(6), 1121–1129.

Mishler, E. G. (1984). *The discourse of medicine: Dialectics of medical interviews.* Norwood: Ablex.

Nairn, R. G. (2007). Media portrayals of mental illness, or is it madness? A review. *Australian Psychologist, 42*(2), 138–146.

Nairn, R., Coverdale, S., & Coverdale, J. H. (2011). A framework for understanding media depictions of mental illness. *Academic Psychiatry, 35*(3), 202–206.

Ng, R. M. (2000). The influence of Confucianism on Chinese conceptions of power, authority, and the rule of law. In D. R. Heisey (Ed.), *Chinese perspectives in rhetoric and communication* (pp. 45–56). Stamford: Ablex.

Olstead, R. (2002). Contesting the text: Canadian media depictions of the conflation of mental illness and criminality. *Sociology of Health and Illness, 24*(5), 621–643.

Pearson, V. (1996). The Chinese equation in mental health policy and practice. *International Journal of Law and Psychiatry, 19*(3/4), 437–458.

Peng, W., & Tang, L. (2010). Health content in Chinese newspapers. *Journal of Health Communication, 15*(7), 695–711.

Phillips, M., Chen, H., Diesfeld, K., Xie, B., Cheng, H., Mellsop, G., & Liu, X. (2013). China's new mental health law: Reframing involuntary treatment. *American Journal of Psychiatry, 170*(6), 588–591.

Qiu, J. L. (2000). Interpreting the Dengist rhetoric of building socialism with Chinese characteristics. In D. R. Heisey (Ed.), *Chinese perspectives in rhetoric and communication* (pp. 249–280). Stamford: Ablex.

Ramsay, G. (2008). *Shaping minds: A discourse analysis of Chinese-language community mental health literature.* Amsterdam: John Benjamins.

Ramsay, G. (2013). *Mental illness, dementia and family in China.* London: Routledge.

Ran, M., Xiang, M., Simpson, P., & Chan, C. L. (2005). *Family-based mental health care in rural China.* Hong Kong: Hong Kong University Press.

Reisigl, M., & Wodak, R. (2009). The Discourse-Historical Approach (DHA). In R. Wodak, & M. Meyer (Eds.), *Methods of critical discourse analysis* (pp. 87–121). London: SAGE.

Rhydderch, D., Krooupa, A. M., Shefer, G., Goulden, R., Williams, P., Thornicroft, A., Rose, D., Thornicroft, G., & Henderson, C. (2016). Changes in newspaper coverage of mental illness from 2008 to 2014 in England. *Acta Psychiatrica Scandinavica, 134*(Suppl. 446), 45–52.

Richardson, J. E. (2007). *Analysing newspapers: An approach from critical discourse analysis.* New York: Palgrave Macmillan.

Roberts, R. (2014). The Confucian moral foundation of socialist model man. *New Zealand Journal of Asian Studies, 16*(1), 23–38.

Rosenberg, A. (2018, 18 June). Hiding my mental illness from my Asian family almost killed me: The silent shame of having a mental illness in a Chinese family. *Vox.* www.vox.com/first-person/2018/6/18/17464574/asian-chinese-community-mental-health-illness

Rowe, R., Tilbury, F., Rapley, M., & O'Ferrall, I. (2003). "About a year before the breakdown I was having symptoms": Sadness, pathology and the Australian newspaper media. *Sociology of Health and Illness, 25*(6), 680–696.

Rukavina, T. V., Nawka, A., Brborović, O., Jovanović, N., Kuzman, M. R., Nawková, L., Bednárová, B., Zŭchová, S., Hrodková, M., & Lattova, Z. (2012). Development of the PICMIN (picture of mental illness in newspapers): Instrument to assess mental illness stigma in print media. *Social Psychiatry and Psychiatric Epidemiology, 4*(7), 1131–1144.

Shepherd, C. (2017, 8 June) China closes 60 celebrity gossip social media accounts. *Reuters.* www.reuters.com/article/us-china-internet-censorship-idUSKBN18Z0J3

Shi-xu. (2014). *Chinese discourse studies.* Hampshire, UK: Palgrave Macmillan.

Shi-xu. (2015). Towards a cultural methodology of human communication research: A Chinese example. In L. Tsung, & W. Wang (Eds.), Contemporary Chinese discourse and social practice in China (pp. 45–58). Amsterdam: John Benjamins.

Suarez, E., & Gadalla, T. M. (2010). Stop blaming the victim: A meta-analysis on rape myths. *Journal of Interpersonal Violence, 25*(11), 2010–2035.

Sun, L., & Zhang, J. (2017). Gender differences among medically serious suicide attempters aged 15–54 years in rural China. *Psychiatry Research, 252*(2017), 57–62.

Tang, L., & Bie, B. (2015). Narratives about mental illnesses in China: The voices of Generation Y. *Health Communication, 31*(2), 171–181.

Thomas, C. (2010). Negotiating the contested terrain of narrative methods in illness contexts. *Sociology of Health and Illness, 32*(4), 647–660.

Thornicroft, A., Goulden, R., Shefer, G., Rhydderch, D., Rose, D., Williams, P., Thornicroft, G., & Henderson, C. (2013). Newspaper coverage of mental illness in England 2008–2011. *British Journal of Psychiatry, 202*(55), s64–s69.

Tian, H. (2012). Discursive production of teaching quality assessment report: A critical discourse analysis. In P. Chilton, H. Tian, & R. Wodak (Eds.), *Discourse and socio-political transformations in contemporary China* (pp. 85–104). Amsterdam: John Benjamins.

Tolton, L. (2009). *Legitimation of violence against women in Colombia: A feminist critical discourse analytic study.* [Doctoral dissertation, The University of Queensland].

Topiwala, A., Wang, X., & Fazel, S. (2012). Chinese forensic psychiatry and its wider implications. *Journal of Forensic Psychiatry and Psychology, 23*(1), 1–6.

van Dijk, T. A. (2000). *Ideology: A multidisciplinary approach.* Thousand Oaks, CA: SAGE.

van Dijk, T. A. (2014). Discourse, cognition, society. In J. Angermuller, D. Maingueneau, & R. Wodak (Eds.), *Discourse Studies reader: Main currents in theory and analysis* (pp. 388–399). Amsterdam: John Benjamins.

van Dijk, T. A. (2015). Critical discourse analysis. In D. Tannen, H. E. Hamilton, & D. Schiffrin (Eds.), *The handbook of discourse analysis* (pp. 466–485). Malden, MA: Wiley Blackwell.

Varshney, M., Mahapatra, A., Krishnan, V., Gupta, R., & Deb, K. S. (2016). Violence and mental illness: What is the true story? *Journal of Epidemiology and Community Health, 70*(3), 223–225.

Wahl, O., Wood, A., & Richards, R. (2002). Newspaper coverage of mental illness: Is it changing? *Psychiatric Rehabilitation Skills, 6*(1), 9–31.

Wang, C. W., Chan, C. L. W., & Yip, P. S. F. (2014). Suicide rates in China from 2002 to 2011: An update. *Social Psychiatry and Psychiatric Epidemiology, 49*(6), 929–941.

Wang, J. (2002). Research on Chinese communication campaigns: A historical review. In W. Jia, X. Lu, & D. R. Heisey (Eds.), *Chinese communication theory and research: Reflections, new frontiers, and new directions* (pp. 131–146). London: Ablex.

Wang, W. (2015). Co-construction of migrant workers' identities on a TV talk show in China. In L. Tsung & W. Wang (Ed.), *Contemporary Chinese discourse and social practice in China* (pp. 125–142). Amsterdam: John Benjamins.

Whitley, R., Adeponle, A., & Miller, A. R. (2015). Comparing gendered and generic representations of mental illness in Canadian newspapers: An exploration of the chivalry hypothesis. *Social Psychiatry and Psychiatric Epidemiology, 50*(2), 325–333.

Whitley, R., & Berry, S. (2013). Trends in newspaper coverage of mental illness in Canada: 2005–2010. *Canadian Journal of Psychiatry, 58*(2), 107–112.

Whitley, R., & Wang, J. W. (2017). Good news? A longitudinal analysis of newspaper portrayals of mental illness in Canada 2005 to 2015. *Canadian Journal of Psychiatry, 62*(4), 278–285.

Xue, L., Shi, Y. W., Knoll, J., & Zhao, H. (2015). Chinese forensic psychiatry: History, development and challenges. *Journal of Forensic Science and Medicine, 1*(1), 61–67.

Yip, K. S. (2007). *Mental health service in the People's Republic of China: Current status and future developments.* New York: Nova Science Publishers.

Zhang, Y., Jin, Y., & Tang, Y. (2015). Framing depression: Cultural and organizational influences on coverage of a public health threat and attribution of responsibilities in Chinese news media, 2000–2012. *Journalism and Mass Communication Quarterly, 92*(1), 99–120.

Zhuang, X. Y., Wong, D. F. K., Cheng, C. W., & Pan, S. M. (2017). Mental health literacy, stigma and perception of causation of mental illness among Chinese people in Taiwan. *International Journal of Social Psychiatry, 63*(6), 498–507.

Appendix

Appendix 1 Key descriptors for *People's Daily* news articles

#	Broad thematic category	Illness name	Headline	Newspaper section	Word count [字]	Date of publ.
1	Celebrity Experience	Severe Mental Illness	Zhang Xinyi, Justin Yuan First Appear Together On Variety Show After Marrying – "Red Braised Pork" Magic Recipe For Conjugal Love [张歆艺袁弘婚后综艺首同框 "红烧肉" 是恩爱法宝]	Entertainment News	407	17/06/16
2	Medicine	Depression	Drop In Range Of Talent (Pay Attention To Problem Of Loss Of "Artisan Spirit") [不拘一格降人才（关注"工匠精神"缺失问题）]	National News	755	07/06/16
3	Medicine	Depression	D-Cal "Proper Exercise Fosters Healthy Growth" Launched In Beijing – Experts Stress Children Should Do Phased Exercise [迪巧:健康成长巧运动在京启动 专家强调儿童应分段运动]	Medical News	650	30/05/16
4	Crime & Civil Law	Depression	"Sichuan Normal University Bloody Murder Case" Suspect Teng Arrested – Previously Identified As Having Depression ["川师大血案"嫌疑人滕某被批捕 此前被鉴定为抑郁症]	National News	215	14/05/16
5	Medicine	Depression	People's Comments On *People's Daily*: Can Daylily Cure TCM's "Depression"? [人民日报人民时评: 黄花菜能治中医的"抑郁"吗？]	Opinion Piece	1028	18/04/16
6	Medicine	Schizophrenia	Schizophrenia Is Prone To Relapse – Needs Early, Ample, Specified Treatment [精神分裂症容易复发 需早期、足疗程规范治疗]	Medical News	1064	14/04/16

(continued)

Appendix 1 (*cont.*)

#	Broad thematic category	Illness name	Headline	Newspaper section	Word count [字]	Date of publ.
7	Celebrity Experience	Severe Mental Illness	Jia Nailiang's 32nd Birthday Party – Li Xiaolu, Tianxin Come On Stage For "Grand Finale" – Revealed Both From Discreetly Wealthy Family Backgrounds [贾乃亮32岁生日会李小璐甜馨"压轴"上台 揭双方家庭背景都是隐形富豪]	Entertainment News	1642	13/04/16
8	Celebrity Experience	Severe Mental Illness	Jia Nailiang Airs Childhood Photos At 32nd Birthday – Song Joong-ki, Eddie Peng, Hu Ge, Wallace Huo – Male Stars' Childhood Photos Dug Up [贾乃亮32岁生日自曝童年照 宋仲基彭于晏胡歌霍建华 男星童年照大扒]	Entertainment News	520	13/04/16
9	Policy	Depression	National People's Congress Representative Wu Xiangdong: Pay Attention To Psychological Health Of Nation's People [全国人大代表吴向东: 关注国民心理健康]	Culinary News	474	14/03/16
10	Policy	Severe Mental Illness	Taiwan Democratic Self-Government League Central Committee Proposal On Strengthening Implementation Of Legal Supervision Work In Compulsory Medical Treatment [台盟中央关于加强强制医疗执行法律监督工作的提案]	Chinese United Front News	1439	29/02/16
11	Suicide	Depression	*People's Daily*: Do Not Ignore Child's Anxiety [人民日报: 别忽视孩子的焦虑]	Opinion Piece	890	29/02/16
12	Celebrity Experience	Depression	Joey Wong Shares Recent Photos Celebrating 49th Birthday – Got Depression? Become Nun? Has Illegitimate Daughter? Rough Lot For Goddess [王祖贤晒近照庆生49岁 得抑郁症? 出家? 有私生女? 看女神坎坷命运]	Entertainment News	2492	01/02/16

#	Category	Theme	Title	News Type	Count	Date
13	Education	Depression	European History, Depression (Global Travelogue) [欧洲史与抑郁症（环球走笔）]	International News	1017	29/01/16
14	Crime & Civil Law	Severe Mental Illness	Sister "Buys" Mentally Ill Brother's Property, Judged Invalid [姐姐"买"下精神病弟弟房产被判无效]	Legal News	690	18/01/16
15	Policy	Severe Mental Illness	Concern Over Dispersal Of Mental Illness Sufferers – How To Resolve This? [精神病人散落之忧如何解]	Medical News	2266	13/01/16
16	Medicine	Severe Mental Illness	Our Nation's Severe Mental Illness Sufferers Reach 4.3 Million [我国严重精神病患者达430万人]	Medical News	769	13/01/16
17	Policy	Severe Mental Illness	Taking Care Of Mental Illness Sufferers – Society Must Not Be "Lax" [照护精神病患，社会别"大撒把"]	Medical News	531	13/01/16
18	Policy	Severe Mental Illness	Nankang, Ganzhou, Buys Medical Insurance For Poverty Relief Recipients [赣州南康为扶贫对象买医保]	National News	358	11/12/15
19	Celebrity Experience	Depression	"Princess Jianning" Rain Lau Contemplated Suicide Due To Depression – In Tears When Hugged By Dicky Cheung ["建宁公主"刘玉翠险因抑郁症轻生 获张卫健拥抱泪崩]	Entertainment News	156	02/11/15
20	Medicine	Depression	Our Nation's Insomnia Rate For Adults Nears 40% – Experts Advise How To Sleep Soundly [我国成年人失眠几率近四成 专家支招如何睡得香]	Medical News	588	29/09/15
21	Crime	Severe Mental Illness	Chinese Student Studying Abroad In USA Gropes Female Students' Thighs At Campus Due To Severe Mental Illness [中国留美学生因精神病在校园乱摸女生大腿]	International News	525	18/09/15
22	Policy	Severe Mental Illness	Shangluo: Works To Rules – Masses Like [商洛：办事规范 群众点赞]	Political News	695	12/09/15

(continued)

Appendix 1 (*cont.*)

#	Broad thematic category	Illness name	Headline	Newspaper section	Word count [字]	Date of publ.
23	Suicide	Depression + Schizophrenia	World Suicide Prevention Day: Impulse Is The Devil – Help You Know About "Impulsive Suicide" [世界预防自杀日：冲动是魔鬼，带你认识"冲动性自杀"]	Medical News	1005	10/09/15
24	Medicine	Depression	Latest Research On "Baby Brain": If Don't Get Depressed, Can Keep Good Memory When Pregnant ["孕傻"最新研究：只要别忧郁 孕期也有好记性]	Science News	515	09/09/15
25	Medicine	Severe Mental Illness	"Acute Transient Psychotic Disorder" Has Precedent In China – Doctors Claim May Be Clinically Misdiagnosed ["急性短暂性精神障碍"国内有先例 医生称临床或会误诊]	Science News	959	08/09/15
26	Medicine	Severe Mental Illness	Chatroom At Your Door (Multiple Perspectives) [家门口有间聊天室（多棱镜）]	National News	1330	07/08/15
27	Art History	Severe Mental Illness	Madness Is God's Gift – "Mentally Abnormal World" In Eyes Of Artists [疯狂是神的礼物 艺术家眼中"精神异常的世界"]	Arts News	1451	28/07/15
28	Celebrity Experience	Depression + Schizophrenia	41-Year-Old Mavis Hee Makes Comeback With Healthy Figure – Current Situation Of Fallen Woman Star Revealed [41岁许美静复出身材发福变型 落魄天后现状揭秘]	Entertainment News	2119	20/07/15
29	Policy	Severe Mental Illness	How Could ¥156 Fix "STD" That ¥310,000 Couldn't Cure? [31万没治好的"性病"咋156元搞定？]	Opinion Piece	1669	15/07/15

30	Suicide	Depression	Chen Lizhi: V-Love Leukaemia Fund – Prolonging As Many Young Lives As Possible [陈砺志：V爱·白血病基金 延续尽可能多的幼小生命]	Charity News	1464	07/07/15
31	Medicine	Depression	Number Of People In Japan Found To Suffer From Psychological Illness Due To Work Hits New High [日本被认定因公罹患心理疾病的人数创新高]	International News	332	26/06/15
32	Medicine	Severe Mental Illness	How Awful Are Drugs?! Shocking Photos Horrifically Compare Before, After Drug Use [毒品到底多可怕？震撼吸毒前后恐怖对比照]	International News	149	25/06/15
33	Policy	Severe Mental Illness	"On Laws" – No Need To Panic About "Compulsory Medical Treatment" [【论法】别提到"强制医疗"就色变]	Medical News	857	17/06/15

Appendix 2 Key descriptors for *Ming Pao* news articles

#	Broad thematic category	Illness name	Headline	Newspaper section	Word count [字]	Date of publ.
34	Crime	Severe Mental Illness	Gunman with Severe Mental Illness Supported Right-Wing Brexit Group [槍手患精神病 撐脫歐右翼團體]	International News	590	18/06/16
35	Crime	Schizophrenia	Crank Calls, Stalked After Work – Male DJs Often Accompany Her Home [致電騷擾等收工 男DJ常護花]	Local News	355	15/06/16
36	Celebrity Experience	Depression	Half-Naked Sammy Leung's Sexy Muscles: The Man Reappears [森美半裸騷肌: 雄風再現]	Entertainment News	197	03/06/16
37	Medicine	Severe Mental Illness	Half Of New Cases Of Severe Childhood Mental Illness Wait More Than A Year [兒童精神病新症半數輪候逾年]	Local News	482	26/05/16
38	Medicine	Depression	Watch Out If Feeling Down For 2 Weeks! [Down足兩星期, 小心！]	Special Column	977	23/05/16
39	Medicine	Depression	UK Research Finds "Magic Mushrooms" Can Treat Depression [英研「迷幻蘑菇」治抑鬱]	International News	414	19/05/16
40	Medicine	Depression + Psychosis	Alcoholics Should Seek Medical Help When Giving Up Drinking [酗酒者戒酒宜找醫護]	Local News	663	16/05/16
41	Suicide	Depression	Having Revealed Worries Over Raising Child, 9-Months Pregnant 19-Year-Old Woman Jumps To Her Death [曾透露擔心如何育兒 懷胎9月 19歲孕婦墮斃]	Local News	657	11/05/16
42	Everyday Personal Experience	Depression	Lonely Boy Played Cello To Comfort Himself, Met Good Teachers – Paid 3 Years' Fees – Offered Half Tuition Waiver [孤獨少年拉琴解愁遇明師 代交3年費用 額減一半學費]	Education News	756	10/05/16

43	Everyday Personal Experience	Schizophrenia	Extra Screening Of "Ten Years" – Hope For Tomorrow! [同場加映：「十年」希望在明天！]	Special Column	1544	08/05/16
44	Crime	Schizophrenia	Retirement Home Involved In Embezzling Mentally Ill Woman's 230,000 HKD – Coaxed Into Signing Investment Contract – Police Refuse Further Investigation [安老院涉吞精神病婦23萬 勸誘簽署投資合約 警拒深入調查]	Local News	1073	07/05/16
45	Crime	Schizophrenia	Attacks Diners With Fake Gun – Schizophrenic Woman Sentenced With Hospitalisation Order [假槍襲食客 精神分裂婦判醫院令]	Local News	266	06/05/16
46	Crime	Severe Mental Illness	Seizes Opportunity To Kiss Face, Has Oral Sex – Pakistani Man Pretends To Ask Directions, Molests 2 Youth [乘機吻臉口交 巴漢扮問路猥褻兩青年]	Local News	466	03/05/16
47	Politics & Activism	Severe Mental Illness	People In Recovery: Social Environment Is More Troublesome [康復者：社會環境更困擾]	Local News	427	03/05/16
48	Politics & Activism	Severe Mental Illness	People With Personal Experience Make Declaration – Hope To Eliminate Misunderstanding About Severe Mental Illness – Resent "Ravings, Weird Behaviour" Remarks By Chris Wat Wing-Yin – Plan To File Complaint With Equal Opportunities Commission [過來人親身發聲 冀消除精神病誤解 不滿屈穎妍「妄語怪行」論 擬平機會投訴]	Local News	955	03/05/16
49	Everyday Personal Experience	Depression	Learn To "Humble Oneself" – Tang How-Kong Walks Away From Depression [學縮細「自我」鄧厚江走出抑鬱]	Local News	300	27/04/16
50	Crime	Severe Mental Illness	Mental Illness Sufferer's Eyes Gouged Out By Ward-Mate [精神病人被病友挖掉雙眼]	Mainland Chinese News	196	24/04/16
51	Politics & Activism	Severe Mental Illness	Francis T. Lui "Cites Expert": Claims Hong Kong Independence Supporters Have Personality Disorder [雷鼎鳴「引述專家」：倡港獨者人格障礙]	Local News	652	22/04/16

(continued)

Appendix 2 *(cont.)*

#	Broad thematic category	Illness name	Headline	Newspaper section	Word count [字]	Date of publ.
52	Crime	Schizophrenia	Mentally Ill Criminal Pretends To Be Scholar – Donated Sperm Bears 36 Descendants [精神病犯冒才子 捐精誕36後代]	International News	545	21/04/16
53	Crime	Depression	Prints, Sells Nearly 1000 MTR Tickets – Station Manager Gets 5 Months Jail [印近千港鐵票出售 站務主任囚5月]	Local News	460	21/04/16
54	Crime	Severe Mental Illness	Woman K-Pop Fan Without Boarding Pass Goes Through 3 Checks, Reaches Boarding Gate [無登機證哈韓女 機場過三關抵登機口]	Local News	758	21/04/16
55	Suicide	Depression + Schizophrenia	Cheung Hing-Yee: Changing Opinion About Suicide Since 90s: Why Do We Have To Be Happy? [張馨儀：90年代至今自殺輿論變遷：為什麼不得不快樂？]	Special Column	2203	16/04/16
56	Celebrity Experience	Schizophrenia	"Star Wars" Child Star Sent To Hospital With Schizophrenia [《星戰》童星患思覺失調送院]	Entertainment News	307	12/04/16
57	Politics & Activism	Severe Mental Illness	Vincent Cheng: Let's Rise Up Against Remarks Defaming Mentally Ill! [鄭仲仁：我們就來起義，反對抹黑精神病人的言論！]	Special Column	880	11/04/16
58	Crime	Schizophrenia	Kitchen Hand Robs 80-Year-Old Woman – Court Petition Reveals Schizophrenia [廚工劫八旬婦 求情揭思覺失調]	Local News	445	08/04/16
59	Crime	Severe Mental Illness	Woman Slaps Son's Teacher Over 10 Times – Gets Suspended Sentence [婦摑兒子教師逾10巴判緩刑]	Local News	511	01/04/16
60	Crime	Severe Mental Illness	Shenzhen Online Uber-Type Taxis Lack Oversight – 1000 Drivers Have Drug Record [深圳網絡召車欠監管 千司機曾涉毒]	Mainland Chinese News	409	31/03/16

61	Celebrity Experience	Depression	Old Photo Of Fat "Prison Break" Male Star Ridiculed – Reveals Overeating During Low Point In Life [《逃》男星脹爆舊照被嘲笑 自揭暴食人生低潮]	Entertainment News	605	30/03/16
62	Crime	Severe Mental Illness	Naked Male Worker Tries To Rape Schoolgirl at School [裸男工校內圖姦女生]	Mainland Chinese News	246	30/03/16
63	Crime	Severe Mental Illness	Fitness Centre Complaint – Autistic Man Pays 90,000 HKD All Up For Membership [指健身中心入會 自閉男前後付9萬]	Local News	453	29/03/16
64	Crime	Depression	Depressed Woman Gets 7 Months Jail For Shoplifting Clothes – Appeals Judge Claims Sentence Too Harsh [抑鬱婦偷衫囚7月 上訴官稱判太重]	Local News	606	22/03/16
65	Suicide	Severe Mental Illness	Education Watcher: Scholars: Put Suicide On Table – Do Your Homework, Don't Just Rely On Intuition / By Yu Chien-Chi [教育線眼：學者：自殺「攤開講」 做足功課忌憑直覺／文：余謙之]	Local News	962	16/03/16
66	Medicine	Severe Mental Illness	Things You Should Know: Strictly Remember "3 No's" To Avoid Upsetting Sufferer [知多啲：緊記「三不」 免刺激患者]	Special Column	502	14/03/16
67	Everyday Personal Experience	Schizophrenia	Taking Care Of Mentally Ill Relative By Yourself – Don't Forget To Take Care Of Yourself To Avoid Breakdown [獨力照料精神病親人 照顧不忘自顧防爆煲]	Special Column	1486	14/03/16
68	Medicine	Severe Mental Illness	Proportion Of Teenagers With Severe Mental Illness Similar To Adults But Receive Far Less Counselling [青少年精神病比率相若 接受輔導遠不及成年人]	Local News	487	13/03/16
69	Suicide	Severe Mental Illness	"Impetuous" 14-Year-Old Twice Attempts Suicide – Guilty About Mother Looking Back – 21-Year-Old Mother Implores Don't Go Head To Head With Children [14歲「衝動」兩度自殺 回首對母愧疚 21歲母籲勿與子女便碰硬]	Local News	659	13/03/16
70	Crime	Severe Mental Illness	Mentally Ill Man Bashes Victim's Head During Robbery – Jailed For 5 Years 9 Months [精神病漢扑頭搶劫 囚5年9月]	Local News	295	11/03/16

(continued)

Appendix 2 (*cont.*)

#	Broad thematic category	Illness name	Headline	Newspaper section	Word count [字]	Date of publ.
71	Crime	Severe Mental Illness	Threw 9-Year-Old Son Against Wall – Hit Head With Rubber Pole – Man With Many Children Admits Child Abuse [掟9歲子攤牆 膠棍打頭 多仔公認虐兒]	Local News	596	11/03/16
72	Crime	Severe Mental Illness	Mentally Ill Man Stabs Passer-By In Neck – Citizen Follows, Helps Arrest [精神病漢刺途人頸 市民跟蹤助拘捕]	Local News	850	09/03/16
73	Suicide	Depression + Severe Mental Illness	Lobo Louie: Opportunities Abound To Make Living In Sports Industry [雷雄德: 運動出路闊 「搵到食」]	Local News	291	08/03/16
74	Crime	Severe Mental Illness	Mentally Ill Man Doubts Fathering Son – Knifes Wife, Son, Sentenced With Hospitalisation Order [疑子非親生 精神病漢斬妻兒判入院令]	Local News	280	02/03/16
75	Everyday Personal Experience	Schizophrenia	Father Sooner Believes Daughter Possessed Than Schizophrenic – Starts To Accept Fact After Getting Medical Help – Lets Go Of Worried Indecision, Firmness, Faces Up Together [父寧信撞邪 不信女兒覺失思覺 求醫後始接受事實 放下徬徨權威同面對]	Local News	884	28/02/16
76	Celebrity Experience	Depression	Fiona Sit Earnestly Thanks Mainland Chinese Fans [薛凱琪內地謝票勁冧粉絲]	Entertainment News	269	27/02/16
77	Crime	Severe Mental Illness	Psychiatric Hospital Patient Chases, Knifes Woman Passer-By – After Assault Wanders Around – Arrested On Return To Rehab Centre [精神病院友追斬女途人 行兇後遊蕩 返復康中心被拘]	Local News	714	27/02/16
78	Crime	Severe Mental Illness	Claims Possessed, Molests Little Girl – Old Man In 60s Sentenced With Hospitalisation Order [稱撞邪猥女童 六旬翁判囚醫院令]	Local News	339	20/02/16

79	Celebrity Experience	Severe Mental Illness	Kate Becomes Guest Editor [凱特客串做編輯]	International News	105	18/02/16
80	Politics & Activism	Severe Mental Illness	Nearly Half Of Middle-Aged People In Recovery From Mental Illness Unemployed – 44% Live Below Poverty Line – HKCSS Urged To Increase Employment Support [中年精神康復者近半失業 44%活在貧窮線下 社聯促增就業支援]	Local News	597	18/02/16
81	Crime	Severe Mental Illness	Attempts Suicide With Wife, Daughter By Burning Charcoal – Mentally Ill Man Accused Of Conspiring To Murder [圖與妻攜女燒炭 精神病漢涉串謀謀殺]	Local News	308	17/02/16
82	Suicide	Severe Mental Illness	Tianjin Inspector Dies Strangely In Corridor [津紀檢官離奇走廊死]	Mainland Chinese News	315	01/02/16
83	Everyday Personal Experience	Depression	Young Mother Suffered From Depression: Tried To Bang Head Against Wall [曾患抑鬱年輕媽媽: 試過撼頭埋牆]	Local News	482	23/01/16
84	Crime	Schizophrenia	Got Severe Mental Illness After Birth Of Daughter – Woman Knifes Husband, Sentenced To Siu Lam Psychiatric Centre [誕女後患精神病 婦斬夫判入小欖]	Local News	461	23/01/16
85	Suicide	Severe Mental Illness	5 Stab Wounds To Body – Dead Woman Probably Self-Harms [身中5刀 倒斃婦疑自殘]	Local News	279	16/01/16
86	Crime	Depression	Father Dead, Mother Depressed, Greedy For Quick Money – Young Drug Dealer Jailed For 13 Years 4 Months [父亡母鬱貪快錢 菁年販毒囚13年4月]	Local News	302	16/01/16
87	Suicide	Severe Mental Illness	Woman Stabbed Multiple Times – Dies in Flat [婦人中多刀倒斃劏房]	Local News	352	15/01/16
88	Crime	Depression	Teacher Allegedly Discloses Exam Questions – Accuses ICAC Officer Of Tricking Verbal Confession [涉洩試題教師 指廉署騙落口供]	Local News	281	14/01/16

(continued)

Appendix 2 (*cont.*)

#	Broad thematic category	Illness name	Headline	Newspaper section	Word count [字]	Date of publ.
89	Everyday Personal Experience	Depression	A Special Child: Tourette Syndrome Experience Becomes Inspiration – Overcomes Life's Difficulties Through Painting [與別不童：妥瑞症經歷化成靈感 畫筆戰勝崎嶇路]	Special Column	1126	12/01/16
90	Celebrity Experience	Depression	Ana R. Reveals Madly Crying Over Daughter – Just Back At Work After Giving Birth [Ana R.自爆為囡囝狂喊 產後首復工]	Entertainment News	379	07/01/16
91	Medicine	Schizophrenia	Traces 1 Year Before Hallucinations Hit – Prelude to Schizophrenia – Memory Loss, Insomnia [幻覺來襲前一年有迹可尋 思覺失調前奏：失憶失眠]	Special Column	1159	04/01/16
92	Suicide	Depression	Uni Student Posts On Microblog – Farewells 2015, Jumps To His Death [大學生發微博告別2015跳樓亡]	Mainland Chinese News	515	02/01/16
93	Everyday Personal Experience	Depression	Psychologist: Story of A-Ching (II): Guardian Angel, Treasure Box, Trains [心理醫生：阿晴的故事（二）：守護小天使、寶盒與火車]	Special Column	2934	27/12/15
94	Celebrity Experience	Depression	Rain Lau: Luckily Scared Of Death – Suffers Depression, Contemplates Suicide [劉玉翠：幸自己驚死 患抑鬱症曾想輕生]	Entertainment News	226	24/12/15
95	Celebrity Experience	Depression	Ruth Chen's New Song Encourages People To Bravely Face Depression [曾路得新歌鼓勵人勇敢面對抑鬱]	Entertainment News	158	24/12/15
96	Politics & Activism	Depression + Severe Mental Illness	A Small Household Appliance – Fulfil Their Christmas Wish [一件小家電 圓他們的聖誕願望]	Local News	373	24/12/15
97	Politics & Activism	Severe Mental Illness	Wong Yee Him: How Is It Mental Illness Sufferers Can Again Be Discriminated Against? [黃以謙：精神病患者豈能再被歧視]	Special Column	1272	22/12/15

Appendix 3 Key descriptors for *Liberty Times* news articles

#	Broad thematic category	Illness name	Headline	Newspaper section	Word count [字]	Date of publ.
98	Crime	Depression	Robs Jewellery Store Holding Kitchen Knife – Depressed Single Mother Arrested [持菜刀搶銀樓 單親憂鬱媽被逮]	Local News	333	20/06/16
99	Crime	Severe Mental Illness	Shot UK Parliamentarian Dead – Killer Hollers In Court [槍殺英議員 兇手出庭叫囂]	Finance News	399	19/06/16
100	Crime	Severe Mental Illness	Younger Brother Slashes Older Brother With Watermelon Knife – Claims To Have Severe Mental Illness [弟拿西瓜刀砍傷兄 供稱精神病]	Local news	233	18/06/16
101	Crime	Depression	Drugs, Sexually Assaults Young Girl – She Jumps Off Building – Sentenced To 10 Years Jail, Fined 1 Million [餵毒性侵害少女跳樓 判10年賠100萬]	Local News	363	18/06/16
102	Medicine	Depression	Home Carers Speak Out – Ganlin To Hold Seminar [家庭照顧者吐心聲 甘霖將辦座談]	Local News	566	16/06/16
103	Medicine	Depression	Taking Care Of Dementia Sufferers, Watch Out For Depression [照顧失智者 小心憂鬱症]	Medical News	598	10/06/16
104	Celebrity Experience	Depression	Young Eli Hsieh Leaps Into The Starlight – Tragically Bullied, Gets Depression [謝震廷年少躍星光 慘遭霸凌患憂鬱症]	Entertainment News	421	10/06/16
105	Everyday Personal Experience	Depression	Different Coloured Fairy Tale – Sleeping Beauty [異色童話館 睡美人]	Special Column	376	05/06/16

(continued)

Appendix 3 *(cont.)*

#	Broad thematic category	Illness name	Headline	Newspaper section	Word count [字]	Date of publ.
106	Crime	Depression	Slaps Foe – Fined 35,000 [甩仇人一巴掌 判賠3萬5]	Local News	483	05/06/16
107	Crime	Depression	Burns Down Ex-Boyfriend's Shop – Woman Sentenced To 10 Years 8 Months Jail [燒前男友店 婦判10年8月]	Local News	161	02/06/16
108	Everyday Personal Experience	Depression	Mother Owes 50 Million Gambling Debt – Daughter Walks Out Of Deep Valley, Becomes Designer [母欠賭債5千萬 女走出幽谷當設計師]	Local News	521	26/05/16
109	Medicine	Depression	Always Grumbling About Pain, Always Forgetful – Be Worried, It Could Be Depression [老喊痛又忘東忘西 恐憂鬱症上身]	Medical News	702	24/05/16
110	Suicide	Depression	Drops 5 Metres Off Suhua Highway Slope – Depressed Motorcyclist's Cause Of Death Awaits Investigation [跌落蘇花公路5米邊坡 憂鬱騎士死因待查]	Local News	455	24/05/16
111	Crime	Severe Mental Illness	Man With Suspected Severe Mental Illness Smashes 16 Cars 2 Days In Succession [疑罹精神病 男2天連砸16車]	Local News	347	18/05/16
112	Politics & Activism	Severe Mental Illness	Homicide, Correctional Rehabilitation & Psychopathology [殺人、教化與精神病理]	Special Column	1442	16/05/16
113	Medicine	Depression	Research Finds Women More Easily Depressed Than Men [研究發現 女比男更易憂鬱]	Medical News	561	13/05/16
114	Suicide	Depression	Couple Takes Pills In Succession – Wife Dies, Husband Saved [夫妻先後吞藥 妻死夫獲救]	Local News	127	13/05/16

115	Politics & Activism	Depression	Prevent Avoiding Military Service By Feigning Illness – Plan To Extend Hospital Observation Period To 4 Weeks [防裝病停役 住院觀察擬延長至 4 週]	Political News	324	13/05/16
116	Celebrity Experience	Depression	Ting Ting Apologises For Touching Female Star – Bao Er, Ga Ga Share Lovers' Attire [廷廷沾女星道歉 寶兒情侶衣挺嫂嗄]	Entertainment News	321	08/05/16
117	Crime	Depression	25-Year-Old Woman Robs Jewellery Store – Wounds 62-Year-Old Woman Right After Getting Bail [25歲女搶銀樓才交保 又殺傷62歲婦]	Local News	315	08/05/16
118	Everyday Personal Experience	Depression	She Gracefully Declines Commendation – Being a Good Mother More True To Heart [她婉拒模範表揚 扮好媽媽角色卡實在]	Lifestyle News	599	05/05/16
119	Medicine	Depression	Dearly Love Mum On Festive Day – Be On Look Out For Old Age Depression [佳節疼媽媽 留心老年憂鬱症]	Local News	552	04/05/16
120	Celebrity Experience	Depression	Carolyn Chen, Debby Yang Wage War On Internet – Patience Has Limits, Hits Back With Pic Giving The Finger [陳珮珊楊琪網路開戰 忍耐有極限回擊中指照]	Medical News	443	30/04/16
121	Celebrity Experience	Depression	Gwyneth Takes New Love To Party Barefoot [葛妮絲赤腳帶新歡參加派對]	Entertainment News	243	26/04/16
122	Medicine	Severe Mental Illness	Psychiatry Boom – Yet Resident Doctor Numbers Drop Year After Year [精神科夯 住院醫師員額卻年年減]	Lifestyle News	682	24/04/16
123	Celebrity Experience	Depression	Ting Ting Gets Away To US, Takes Pic With Cutie – Magic Power 3 Scared Out Of Wits By Prank In Okinawa [廷廷飛美散心合影美眉 MP3沖繩搞嚇鬼破膽]	Entertainment News	392	23/04/16
124	Celebrity Experience	Depression	Magic Power's Ting Ting Discloses Depression Treatment To Last 6 More Months [MP廷廷自揭憂鬱療程再用半年]	Entertainment News	345	20/04/16

(continued)

Appendix 3 *(cont.)*

#	Broad thematic category	Illness name	Headline	Newspaper section	Word count [字]	Date of publ.
125	Medicine	Schizophrenia	Receive Treatment, Take Medication On Time – Schizophrenia Sufferers Won't Cause Trouble [接受治療 定期服藥 思覺失調患者不使壞]	Medical News	603	16/04/16
126	Medicine	Depression	Changing LED Light Spectrum Can Relieve Depression [改變LED燈光譜 可舒緩憂鬱症]	Lifestyle News	560	14/04/16
127	Crime	Depression	Signs "Cheng Chieh Fan Club" – Sentenced To Jail For Sending Threatening Text [署名鄭傑後援會 寄恐嚇信判刑]	Local News	269	13/04/16
128	Celebrity Experience	Schizophrenia	*Star Wars* Child Star Bullied Due To Fame – Tragically Gets Schizophrenia [星戰童星爆紅遭霸凌 慘得精神分裂]	Entertainment News	295	12/04/16
129	Politics & Activism	Severe Mental Illness	Psychiatrist: Strengthen Social Safety Net – Should Give More Power To Social Workers [精神科醫師: 健全社會安全網 應強化社工權力]	Special Column	549	11/04/16
130	Celebrity Experience	Depression	Ting Ting Finds It Hard To Shake Off Depression, Leaves Band – Magic Power 6 Missing 3, Comeback Open-Ended [廷廷難甩憂鬱離團 MP6缺3復出無期]	Entertainment News	677	09/04/16
131	Suicide	Depression	Suffers From Depression – Woman Hairdresser Jumps Off Building To Her Death [罹患憂鬱症 女美髮師墜樓亡]	Local News	224	06/04/16
132	Politics & Activism	Severe Mental Illness	Forcibly Put "Shaky Bro" In Hospital – KP Attacked For Trampling On Human Rights [強制「搖搖哥」送醫 柯P被轟踐踏人權]	Lifestyle News	827	02/04/16
133	Politics & Activism	Severe Mental Illness	Forced Hospitalisation Determinations – Police, Fire Officers Mystified [強制送醫醫認定 警、消茫然]	Local News	501	01/04/16

134	Crime	Depression	"If Child Murder Case Gets Light Sentence, I Will Do The Same!" – Man Arrested For Drunken Ravings [「殺童案輕判就模仿」男醉後狂言被逮]	Local News	242	31/03/16
135	Politics & Activism	Severe Mental Illness	Child Killer Suspect Mentally Ill? Politician Criticises Criminal Investigation Division, Fears Will Help Killer Get Off [殺童嫌精神病？議員批刑大恐幫脫罪]	Local News	285	31/03/16
136	Politics & Activism	Schizophrenia	Prevent Community Incidents – KP: Neighbourhood Groups Important [防社會事件 柯P：鄰里組織重要]	Local News	343	31/03/16
137	Politics & Activism	Schizophrenia	Nationalist Party Caucus Calls For Increased School Security [國民黨議會黨團 要求加強校安]	Local News	343	31/03/16
138	Politics & Activism	Severe Mental Illness	Police Float Killer Mentally Ill – Doctor Forthrightly Says Too Arbitrary [警定調兇手是精障 醫師直言太武斷]	Local News	675	30/03/16
139	Crime	Depression	Cuts Cleaner With Saw – Says Wants To Save Cockroaches [鋸殺清潔員 說要救蟑螂]	Political News	439	30/03/16
140	Everyday Personal Experience	Severe Mental Illness	Woman Saves Change Bit By Bit – Resolute As Anonymous Donor To Family Care [婦點滴存零錢 堅當無名氏捐家扶]	Local News	553	27/03/16
141	Medicine	Depression	Seem To Be Breaking Out With Every Illness – In Fact It's SAPHO Syndrome [看似百病叢生 其實是皮膚關節症候群]	Medical News	711	26/03/16
142	Suicide	Depression	Woman With Depression, Bipolar Disorder Tries To Jump Off Building, Stopped [女患憂鬱及躁鬱症 欲跳樓遭制止]	Local News	136	26/03/16
143	Medicine	Depression	Crazy Online Shopping – High School Girl Has Depression [瘋狂網購 高中女罹憂鬱症]	Local News	443	24/03/16

(continued)

Appendix 3 *(cont.)*

#	Broad thematic category	Illness name	Headline	Newspaper section	Word count [字]	Date of publ.
144	Crime	Depression	9-Year-Old Sexually Assaulted By Mother's De-Facto – Suffers 14 Years, Lecher Arrested [9歲遭母同居人性侵 痛苦14年逮狼]	Local News	456	23/03/16
145	Crime	Schizophrenia	Strikes, Throws Faeces, Sets Fire, Inundates – Mentally Ill Man Found Not Guilty [打人潑糞、火攻水淹 精障男判無罪]	Local News	296	23/03/16
146	Everyday Personal Experience	Severe Mental Illness	Life's Work Book – Her Days In The Psychiatric Ward [人生作業簿 她在精神病房的日子]	Special Column	801	20/03/16
147	Celebrity Experience	Depression	Claudia Wu Confides In Tears – Ex-Husband Demands 500,000 [吳玟萱淚訴 遭前夫討50萬]	Entertainment News	247	20/03/16
148	Everyday Personal Experience	Schizophrenia	Helping Each Other In Illness – Schizophrenic Mother, Daughter Fight Serious Disease [疾病相扶持 思覺失調母女抗病魔]	Local News	479	19/03/16
149	Everyday Personal Experience	Severe Mental Illness	Life In The Nursing Station – Black Sheep [人生護理站 黑羊]	Special Column	666	18/03/16
150	Crime	Schizophrenia	"Go Kill Someone!" – Schizophrenic Man Allegedly Hears Voices, Stabs Aunt To Death, Charged [「快去殺人」 思覺失調男疑幻聽刺死姑姑被訴]	Local News	404	18/03/16
151	Suicide	Depression	Daxi Charred Corpse Shock – Depressed Woman Self-Immolates [大溪駭見焦屍 憂鬱婦自焚]	Local News	239	16/03/16

No.			Title			
152	Everyday Personal Experience	Depression	Refuses To Abort Daughter Under One-Child Policy – Single Mother Goes Back To Taiwan, Sells Sweet Potatoes [拒一胎化殺女 單親媽媽回台賣地瓜]	Lifestyle News	557	16/03/16
153	Crime	Depression	Report On Germanwings Air Crash Just Released – Co-Pilot Deliberately Crashed Into Mountain [德翼空難報告出爐 副機師蓄意撞山]	International News	218	14/03/16
154	Crime	Depression	Takes Illicit Drugs To Treat Depression – Entire Building Filled With Strange Odour [吸毒治憂鬱 整棟大樓飄怪味咪]	Local News	166	13/03/16
155	Suicide	Depression	Suicide Woman Jammed Dead In 20cm Space Between Buildings [20公分大樓縫 卡死輕生婦]	Local News	227	12/03/16
156	Crime	Depression	No Experience! On Hearing Jewellery Store Sound Police Alarm, Woman Robber Just Stands There Bemused [沒經驗聽到銀樓報警 女搶匪愣住]	Local News	356	11/03/16
157	Suicide	Depression	Young Daughter Missing 2 Years – Police Officer Bemoans Colleagues Can't Help [幼女失蹤兩年 員警嘆警友幫不上忙]	Local News	446	06/03/16
158	Crime	Depression	Dark AV Sector – Japanese Girls Forced To Make Film [暗黑AV界 日女遭強迫拍片]	International News	663	05/03/16
159	Medicine	Depression	Menopausal Upheaval – Woman Get Depression, Insomnia [更年期來亂 婦憂鬱又失眠]	Medical News	533	04/03/16
160	Celebrity Experience	Depression	Commemorating Comic Master – Tunnel Named After Robin Williams [緬懷喜劇大師 隧道取名實威廉斯]	Entertainment News	217	03/03/16
161	Celebrity Experience	Depression	Shennio Lin Releases Album After 12 Years – Tearful Over Parents' Presence [林忝儀等12年發片 父母站台秒飆淚]	Entertainment News	268	02/03/16

(continued)

Appendix 3 *(cont.)*

#	Broad thematic category	Illness name	Headline	Newspaper section	Word count [字]	Date of publ.
162	Everyday Personal Experience	Depression	Music Therapy – Kind Man Plays Piano At Hospital As Volunteer [音樂療癒 暖男當志工到醫院彈琴]	Local News	489	02/03/16
163	Medicine	Depression	Large Temperature Difference – Watch Out For Seasonal Depression [溫差大 小心季節性憂鬱症]	Medical News	465	01/03/16
164	Celebrity Experience	Depression	Irene Chen – Depression, Hair Loss, Failed Marriage – Regrets Being Artist [陳艾琳憂鬱鬼剃頭 婚姻失敗悔當藝人]	Entertainment News	557	01/03/16
165	Suicide	Depression	Depressed Man Tries To Lie On Railway Tracks – Quick-Witted Police Officer Placates Him, Drags Him Back [鬱男欲臥軌 機智警安撫拉回]	Local News	116	01/03/16
166	Everyday Personal Experience	Depression	Husband Accompanies Cancer Wife As Volunteer – 16 Years Loving Companions [夫伴癌妻當志工 16年愛相隨]	Local News	503	01/03/16
167	Suicide	Depression	Woman With Heavy Makeup Attempts Suicide – Thwarted By Police Near Drain [婦濃妝尋短 警大排前攔阻]	Local News	407	29/02/16
168	Politics & Activism	Depression	Hua Kuang Relocation Elegy – 3 Years, 10 Elderly People Die [華光搬遷悲歌 3年10老人過世]	Local News	548	26/02/16
169	Suicide	Depression	Woman Jumps Off Building, Falls Head First Into Car – Dies, Car Written Off [女跳樓栽車內 人亡車報廢]	Local News	200	24/02/16
170	Suicide	Depression	2nd Grade Junior High Schoolboy Jumps To Death Off Building – Family Donates Organs, Helps Others [國二男跳樓亡 家人器捐遺愛]	Local News	184	24/02/16

171	Medicine	Depression	Students With Insomnia, Diarrhoea Before Exams – Anxiety Attack, Relieve Stress Right Away [考生失眠拉肚子 焦慮上身快紓壓]	Medical News	558	22/02/16
172	Celebrity Experience	Depression	Ga Ga's Fancy Pants Girl Posts To Cheer Up Irene Chen [嘎嘎花褲妹發文 對陳艾琳打氣]	Entertainment News	314	18/02/16
173	Celebrity Experience	Depression	Boy Band "51" Goes Past Depression – Engrossed In Jade Design [男團51走過憂鬱 醉心翡翠設計]	Entertainment News	327	16/02/16
174	Celebrity Experience	Depression	Ah Xiang Leaves Band Without Warning – Magic Power Trapped In Split Up Crisis [阿翔無預警退團 MP陷解散危機]	Entertainment News	538	14/02/16
175	Celebrity Experience	Depression	"51" "Enjoy The Moment" Concert – Abin Fang Lends Support [51「及時行樂」開唱 方炯鑌力挺]	Entertainment News	293	06/02/16
176	Medicine	Depression	Latest US Research – Psoriasis Sufferers More Likely Get Depression [美國最新研究 乾癬病患較憂鬱]	Medical News	442	31/01/16
177	Medicine	Depression	Always Complaining About Feeling Unwell – Be Worried, It Could Be Depression, Not Wear & Tear [老是抱怨不舒服 恐憂鬱非退化]	Medical News	424	29/01/16
178	Celebrity Experience	Depression	Magic Power's Ting Ting Has Depression – Posts Farewell, Leaves People Worried [MP廷廷憂鬱症 發文見令人憂]	Entertainment News	332	27/01/16
179	Medicine	Depression	Sin-Lau Oral Cavity Cancer Treatment – Multifaceted Integration Recognised [新樓口腔癌治療 多元整合獲肯定]	Local News	554	27/01/16
180	Celebrity Experience	Depression	Boy Band "51" Rehearses Hard For Concert – Reunion Dinner With Jonathon Lee Unforgettable [51男團為開唱勤操練 難忘李宗盛的團圓飯]	Entertainment News	313	26/01/16

(continued)

Appendix 3 (*cont.*)

#	Broad thematic category	Illness name	Headline	Newspaper section	Word count [字]	Date of publ.
181	Celebrity Experience	Depression	Eli Hsieh Sings Solo While Ill – Jacky Chen, Shuo Hsiao Cheer Him On [謝震廷抱病辦個唱 陳建瑋蕭賀碩捧場]	Entertainment News	202	26/01/16
182	Crime	Depression	Causes Girlfriend To Suicide – Dentist Gets Off Sexual Assault – 1 Year Jail For Grievous Bodily Harm [害女友歐生牙醫性侵脫罪 傷害囚1年]	Local News	463	26/01/16
183	Everyday Personal Experience	Depression	Chao Shih-Yi: Charitable Enterprises Must Be Self-Sufficient [趙士懿: 社企要自己養活自己]	Finance News	783	25/01/16
184	Crime	Depression	Wife Fails To Fix PC – Horror Husband First Beats Then Burns Her [妻修不好電腦 恐怖丈夫先揍後燒]	Local News	542	24/01/16
185	Everyday Personal Experience	Severe Mental Illness	Life In The Nursing Station – Psychiatric Ward [人生護理站 精神病房]	Lifestyle News	390	23/01/16
186	Suicide	Depression	Woman's Corpse In Burnt-Out Car – Probably Jaded From Long Illness, Self-Immolates [火燒車見女屍 疑久病厭世自焚]	Local News	165	23/01/16
187	Crime	Schizophrenia	Rips Up Ballot Paper – Schizophrenic Man Taken Away [撕毀選票 思覺失調症男遭送辦]	Local News	394	17/01/16
188	Politics & Activism	Depression	Stranger Than Politics – Wants To Build Interstellar Theme Park [政見比怪 要蓋星際公園]	Local News	472	15/01/16
189	Crime	Depression	Dead Prisoner Case – Control Yuan Corrects Taipei, Other Prisons [受刑人死亡案 監察院糾正北監等]	Local News	388	14/01/16

190	Medicine	Depression	Aggrieved Kids At School – Doctor: Parents, Don't Disregard It [孩子在校受委屈 醫師: 家長勿輕忽]	Local News	598	14/01/16
191	Celebrity Experience	Depression	Yang Pei-An Once Attempted Suicide – Realises Live In The Moment [楊培安曾輕生 頓悟活在當下]	Entertainment News	314	13/01/16
192	Suicide	Depression	Jen-Wu Home Catches Fire – Man Incinerated [仁武民宅起火 男葬身火窟]	Local News	139	13/01/16
193	Crime	Depression	Dislikes SM Sex Worker – Client To Text Her Children, Forces Her To Submit [搞SM嫌棄 嫖客電告她兒女逼就範]	Local News	304	13/01/16
194	Crime	Depression	Insults Subordinate As Shit For Brains – Hsinchu Science Park Manager Fined 50,000 [罵部屬頭腦裝屎 竹科經理判賠5萬]	Finance News	713	13/01/16
195	Missing Person	Depression	Woman Gets Lost While Driving – Pingtung Police Take Her Back [女開車迷途 屏東警送回]	Local News	166	10/01/16
196	Suicide	Depression	Holds Knife, Forces Wife To Buy Charcoal – Man Attempts Suicide, Rescued [持刀逼妻買炭 男輕生獲救]	Local News	135	09/01/16
197	Finance	Severe Mental Illness	"Ups, Downs Of Taiwan Stocks" – Where Is 2nd OBI Pharma? [<台股青紅燈>浩鼎第二在哪裡?]	Finance News	564	08/01/16
198	Celebrity Experience	Depression	Andy Lau's Healthy Blessing – Boy Band "51" Casts Off Death, Optimistically Moves On [華仔健康喊話 男團「51」甩掉死神樂觀向前]	Entertainment News	374	05/01/16
199	Crime	Depression	Hard To Move On From Love & Money – Woman Sets Fire To Ex-Husband's House [情債錢債難了 女到前夫家縱火]	Local News	625	03/01/16
200	Suicide	Depression	Adult Daughter Wants To Live In Sin – Heartbroken Mother Nearly Jumps In River [女兒大了想同居 傷心母險跳河]	Local News	356	30/12/15

(continued)

Appendix 3 *(cont.)*

#	Broad thematic category	Illness name	Headline	Newspaper section	Word count [字]	Date of publ.
201	Suicide	Depression	Suicides By Drinking Poison With Daughter – Single Mother Coma Index 8 [攜女喝毒液輕生 單親媽昏迷指數8]	Local News	270	30/12/15
202	Missing Person	Depression	New Mother Missing 1 Week – 3–400 Kind-Hearted People Search Mountain [產婦失蹤1週 3、400人熱心搜山]	Local News	524	27/12/15
203	Medicine	Depression	Senior Crisis – Watch Out For Old Age Depression [銀髮族危機 小心老年憂鬱症]	Medical News	633	24/12/15
204	Crime	Depression	Illicit Drugs Hidden In Umbrella Handle – Still Caught By Police [毒藏傘柄 仍被警方查獲]	Local News	192	24/12/15
205	Suicide	Depression	Probably Jaded From Long Illness – Driver Soaked In Petrol Self-Immolates, Dies [疑久病厭世 運將淋油自焚亡]	Local News	371	23/12/15

Index

Printed in the United States
By Bookmasters